MARCHING TOWARD COVERAGE

MARCHING TOWARD COVERAGE

HOW WOMEN CAN LEAD THE FIGHT FOR UNIVERSAL HEALTHCARE

· · · · · · · · · ·

ROSEMARIE DAY

BEACON PRESS, BOSTON

BEACON PRESS
Boston, Massachusetts
www.beacon.org

Beacon Press books
are published under the auspices of
the Unitarian Universalist Association of Congregations.

23 22 21 20   8 7 6 5 4 3 2 1

This book is printed on acid-free paper that meets the uncoated paper
ANSI/NISO specifications for permanence as revised in 1992.

Text design and composition by Kim Arney

The Audre Lorde quote is printed here by permission.

Library of Congress Cataloging-in-Publication Data

Names: Day, Rosemarie, author.
Title: Marching toward coverage : how women can lead the fight for
universal healthcare / Rosemarie Day.
Description: Boston : Beacon Press, [2020] | Includes bibliographical references and index.
Identifiers: LCCN 2019035131 (print) | LCCN 2019035132 (ebook) |
ISBN 9780807018934 (trade paperback) | ISBN 9780807018958 (ebook)
Subjects: LCSH: Health care reform—United States. | Medical policy—
United States. | Women social reformers—United States.
Classification: LCC RA395.A3 D393 2020 (print) | LCC RA395.A3 (ebook) |
DDC 362.10973—dc23
LC record available at https://lccn.loc.gov/2019035131
LC ebook record available at https://lccn.loc.gov/2019035132

*To my family, and to all the women who struggle
to keep their families and communities healthy*

. . . . .

Everyone who is born holds dual citizenship, in the kingdom of the well and in the kingdom of the sick. Although we all prefer to use only the good passport, sooner or later each of us is obliged, at least for a spell, to identify ourselves as citizens of that other place.

—SUSAN SONTAG, "Illness as Metaphor"

I am not free while any woman is unfree, even when her shackles are very different from my own.

—AUDRE LORDE

CONTENTS

PREFACE

WHY DOES OUR HEALTHCARE SYSTEM FAIL SO MANY? And more importantly, what can we do about it? Thousands of people die each year in the US because they don't have health insurance. Many more can't afford their care and are at risk of losing their coverage every single day. Even though the US is one of the richest countries in the world, our citizens are denied the level of access to healthcare that other, less wealthy countries guarantee to theirs.

Adding insult to injury, the numbers show that this burden is disproportionately carried by women. Women are typically responsible for making up to 80 percent of healthcare decisions for their families, and are often caring for their children and elderly parents simultaneously. Even though this means women are likely to have the greatest amount of experience with the healthcare system, we are often subtly guided away from raising our voices, and may feel hesitant about political involvement.

In the wake of the 2016 election and the rise of the #MeToo movement, many Americans—especially women—are growing angrier. I am certainly one of them. As a mother of three with aging parents, and a person at risk of losing coverage if preexisting conditions are no longer protected under the law, the issue of healthcare hits especially close to home for me. With so many others, I have marched, I have fumed, and I have strategized. Ultimately, I decided to write this book.

As with any complex issue, I've found that it's easier to describe problems than to develop answers. With over two decades of experience implementing new healthcare programs and advising healthcare leaders on best practices, I know that fixing the US healthcare system is an enormous task. Fortunately, while marching alongside hundreds of thousands of women as part of the Women's March on Washington in 2017, I had a big "aha" moment: I realized that if we could harness this energy and build on it, we could create a movement to make healthcare a right in the US.

I wrote this book to empower you to do just that, by bringing together two key components: knowledge and activism. I know that life is terribly busy and you may not be able to read the entire book. That's OK! Read some now, save some for later. Some parts may be more important to you now than others. I hope the book, taken as a whole, informs and inspires you.

This is a book about transforming our healthcare coverage system, with feminism as the lens and women as the drivers. The American people have been pushing for better access to healthcare for decades—now is the time to put the pressure on. Now is the time to march. In difficult times, I take solace in one of my favorite quotes from Dr. Martin Luther King Jr.: "The arc of the moral universe is long, but it bends towards justice." In the realm of healthcare, the quote has been modified to suggest that "the arc of the healthcare universe is long, but it bends toward coverage."[1]

But the arc won't bend by itself. Together, we have the power to make change if we join forces and act. Please join me as we keep marching toward coverage.

■ ■ ■ ■ ■ ■

CHAPTER 1

WHY COVERAGE MATTERS

A leader takes people where they want to go. A great leader takes
people where they don't necessarily want to go, but ought to be.

—ROSALYNN CARTER, former First Lady[1]

IN 2017, HEALTHCARE ISSUES HIT ME HARD. My eighty-year-old mother fell,
was hospitalized, had surgery, and was diagnosed with a serious illness.
My eighteen-year-old daughter suffered terrible stomach pains and ongoing
weakness that turned out to be celiac disease. And in the middle of all that,
I discovered I had breast cancer and had to seek treatment. I was stunned.
It felt like things were spiraling out of control. I wanted desperately to help
my mother and daughter. My doctors were telling me to take care of myself.

Each of those issues required a tremendous amount of engagement with
the healthcare system, including numerous visits with physicians, surgeons,
and specialists. However, as difficult as that year was, I found myself continually grateful—not only because the three of us received the care we needed,
but also because, first and foremost, we were able to access that care. My
daughter and I were covered by our family's workplace insurance plan. My
mother was covered by Medicare. Since we all had health insurance coverage, we could focus on getting better and returning to living our lives,
without the nerve-wracking worry about whether we could afford our care
and treatments.

Millions of Americans aren't as fortunate.

As I write this in 2019, approximately twenty-eight million Americans
are uninsured. That's 12 percent of the population under the age of sixty-
five, and the number is starting to grow. Millions more are underinsured,
worrying that the coverage they have isn't enough, or that they might lose
it entirely.[2]

Who are these people? We all know someone. The thirty-something who wants to leave her job to start her own business but won't, because she can't afford nongroup (individual) health insurance. The newlyweds who just discovered that they're going to have a baby but aren't sure if their policy covers maternity care. The forty-year-old who can't get the mental health treatment she needs because her insurance doesn't cover it. The fifty-year-old who's putting off getting a cancer follow-up test because she doesn't have the money to pay the deductible. And all of the people, now including my daughter and me, who may be vulnerable to losing coverage because of their preexisting conditions. The list goes on and on, and if it hasn't happened directly to you, odds are you know someone who's been concerned about their healthcare access. Inadequate access to healthcare is a common and persistent national headache—and in many ways, the pain is suffered mostly by women.

Think about it. Women are more likely to be caregivers for children and elderly parents, and they're more likely to be patients themselves. This means that women are the ones who interact with the healthcare system most often and most intimately. In fact, according to the US Department of Labor, women make approximately 80 percent of all healthcare decisions for their families.[3] As a result, underinsurance and skyrocketing medical costs represent more than a national health crisis; they're a civil rights issue, and the next battlefront for the feminist movement.

Women are serving as the chief medical officers of their families.[4] In the business world, CMOs (or any other kinds of "chiefs") can have enormous influence, especially because they tend to wield massive purchasing power. But as the CMO of a family unit, a woman's influence and purchasing power are quite limited. Most treat healthcare problems as strictly personal or private family issues, instead of recognizing their problems with health coverage as part of a larger systemic failure. So instead of sharing knowledge and resources and organizing to influence policy decisions, women end up struggling alone against a system that's too big and too broken to be affected by their individual concerns. If we were able to harness the power of tens of millions of household CMOs collectively in the political and business arenas, we could expand and improve healthcare access, creating a better world for ourselves, our families, and our nation.

As someone with a passion for public policy who has led change in state government, I have been working to expand access to healthcare coverage for much of my career. Even so, by the end of 2017, my eyes were opened in new ways and my commitment to healthcare reform had deepened profoundly. Not only had I faced my own medical challenges, but over the course of that year, the debate around America's health insurance system became so contentious that I just wasn't able to ignore the turmoil it was causing—personally or professionally. I'll never forget those images I first saw on Twitter one evening in early 2017; it had already been a long day, and then there it was—an all-male group sitting around the White House conference table discussing how to repeal the Affordable Care Act (ACA).[5] Such a move would have far-reaching implications for women, including the elimination of the requirement for maternity coverage. I still recall the anger I felt in that moment, and the frustration that continued building all year, every time more reasonable policy alternatives failed to gain traction.

I emerged from that year more resolved than ever to answer the questions I've been tackling since I started working on social welfare issues in the 1990s. Questions like: How can we make this more fair? How can we improve our healthcare system so that we have fewer disparities and everyone can get the quality care they need? Is access to healthcare enough? What else will help to improve our health? Why can every other developed nation in the world have universal healthcare and better outcomes? And finally, who has the power and the resources necessary to influence our system?

To begin tackling these questions, I delved into our country's history to see whether universal coverage had been considered in the past and if so, why we didn't get there. Access to healthcare is an enormously important national issue that people have been working on for decades. In general terms, healthcare gets a lot of attention because it's close to 20 percent of our national economy, and it affects every single one of us at some point. Despite this, and despite America's status as one of the wealthiest nations in the world, we've never managed to establish a healthcare system that covers every citizen. Surprisingly, there have been only two major points of progress in the effort to expand healthcare access throughout the nation.

First, on July 30, 1965, President Lyndon Johnson signed the Social Security Amendments, establishing Medicare and Medicaid and promising that they would "improve a wide range of health and medical services for Americans of all ages."[6] These programs for the elderly and the poor are still in place today. In fact, they've significantly expanded coverage over the past fifty years, one step at a time.

Forty-five years later, on March 23, 2010, President Barack Obama signed the ACA into law. This second major point of progress for improving healthcare access, nicknamed "Obamacare," is a landmark piece of legislation that impacts a broad spectrum of the healthcare system and sets national standards for health insurance. It's credited with expanding high-quality healthcare coverage to over twenty million Americans. However, it fell short of ensuring that coverage would be affordable for all. Before I dive deeper into the problems of healthcare coverage in the US and identify any solutions, let's take a step back and briefly review some basics, including how insurance works.

HOW HEALTH INSURANCE WORKS

Unless you are independently wealthy—and most of us aren't—you need health insurance to cover your healthcare costs, especially those that would accumulate if you were to suffer from a catastrophic event (a serious injury, a heart attack, a cancer diagnosis, etc.). In fact, one of the leading causes of bankruptcies in the United States involves a medical care need or crisis. Some of it is due to healthcare expenses; some is due to lost time at work. And it's worse for people who don't have health insurance or who have insurance with high cost-sharing. When people without health insurance suffer from a catastrophic health event, they have to pay for their care somehow. Often they put the expenses on their credit cards. Once they've maxed out that option, many go bankrupt.[7]

Health insurance protects people from catastrophic expenses in the same way that other forms of insurance do: it protects individuals financially by sharing risk with a larger group. Health insurance combines groups of people into "risk pools" into which they pay a monthly fee called a "premium." In addition to using monthly premiums, insurers share risk with insured people by charging them other sorts of fees, like co-payments to cover a portion of the costs incurred at the doctor's office. They can also establish "deductibles," the amount people have to pay before the insurer will start to cover any medical costs. All of these fees and forms of cost-sharing are set so that insurers will have enough funds to cover the people who have an expensive healthcare need and are based on the odds that most people won't have a costly need in any given year.

Since no one person can know what may happen to them, it makes sense for each of us to have insurance coverage, just in case we need medical treatment. And because the odds are low that everyone in the risk pools will get sick or injured at once, the more people you have in a risk pool, the better. But even without experiencing the nightmare of a catastrophic event, you benefit since health insurance in the US covers routine doctor's visits and other forms of preventive care, all of which can keep you healthy and relieve suffering, and may even save your life. Having regular checkups with health-care professionals can help you to identify and manage chronic conditions such as diabetes or find a skin cancer before it spreads.

In the US, health insurance is the key to accessing our healthcare system. As many of us know from personal experience, when you show up in the emergency room, one of the first questions is, "What kind of insurance coverage do you have?" And while it may be possible for some people to afford the payments for routine checkups without having health insurance, the minute an emergency arises, or the doctor prescribes a treatment plan, the out-of-pocket costs can skyrocket. Even with health insurance, the out-of-pocket costs can be prohibitively high for many people.

In short, having affordable, high-quality health insurance matters. And it goes far beyond providing financial protection—it's actually a life or death issue. It turns out that people without health insurance are more than six times as likely as the insured to go without needed care due to cost. And, they are at a 3 percent to 41 percent increased risk of death.[8]

THE PATCHWORK QUILT OF COVERAGE

Despite the critical importance of health insurance, Americans, unlike the citizens of all other wealthy countries, do not have universal coverage. Instead, our system of coverage is more like a patchwork quilt—a crazy quilt, even—with no discernible pattern.

Figure 1.1 illustrates a quick picture of health insurance coverage in the US.

As you can see, close to half of the population (49 percent) has health insurance through their (or a family member's) job. The next biggest share of the population (21 percent) has coverage through the Medicaid program, which is for low-income and medically needy people. The remaining pieces of the coverage quilt include Medicare, the program for people age sixty-five and over plus many persons with significant disabilities, covering 14 percent of the population; the "nongroup" or "individual" insurance market, for people buying coverage on their own, which accounts for 6 percent of the population; and other publicly funded programs, such as coverage by the military, which covers 1 percent of the population. The remaining 9 percent have no insurance coverage.

What this figure doesn't show is how your coverage could change over time. Even if you are in one coverage category today, the odds are high that

FIGURE 1.1 Health Insurance Coverage in the US

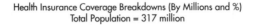

Health Insurance Coverage Breakdowns (By Millions and %)
Total Population = 317 million

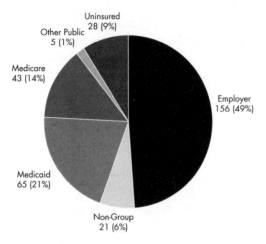

Uninsured
28 (9%)

Other Public
5 (1%)

Medicare
43 (14%)

Employer
156 (49%)

Medicaid
65 (21%)

Non-Group
21 (6%)

Source: "Health Insurance Coverage of the Total Population," Kaiser Family Foundation, last updated 2019, https://www.kff.org.

you will move through different categories over the course of your lifetime. You might have insurance from your employer right now, but if someday you want to quit your job and start your own business, you will likely have to buy your coverage through the individual market. Or, if someday your income is low enough or your health needs are great enough, you may qualify for Medicaid. And when you reach sixty-five years old, as most of us will, you will be able to join Medicare. Because of these dynamics, the numbers of people who move through each coverage category in any given year is much higher than those shown in the graph here. This changing coverage status increases the complexity and uncertainty of healthcare for many Americans.

The other thing this figure doesn't show is the tremendous variation in the types of insurance coverage within most of these categories—the coverage ranges from thick and robust ("platinum" plans) to thin and threadbare (short-term plans). Some coverage includes families; other insurance is just for individuals. This variation is what makes the coverage quilt truly "crazy"; it's not even made up of the same material components all the way across.

These coverage variations are driven largely by the lack of affordability of health insurance for most people, and contrast greatly with how things work in other countries. Our peer nations provide at least some form of basic health coverage (think fleece blanket—simple, warm, and stretchy) to all of their citizens, regardless of age, income, or employment status. In fact, they treat healthcare as a right. They also invest more heavily in social supports. And the results are striking: their populations are healthier and live longer than people in the US do.

And of course, behind every one of those US coverage categories is a real person. This was brought home to me years ago, when I learned that my children's preschool teacher had no health insurance because the preschool, which was a nonprofit serving many low-income members of the community, simply didn't have the revenue to fund that benefit. And she couldn't afford to buy health insurance, given her low salary. Her children qualified for Medicaid, but she was left out in the cold. Here was a working mother who had no coverage and therefore no access to checkups, or any of the care she needed. She was working hard, helping children, and we couldn't afford to cover her. If healthcare were a right, our preschool teacher would have been covered.

If healthcare were a right and we had universal coverage, as well as social supports, then our emotional burdens would be lessened, fewer people would suffer, and more people would live. More people would have the freedom to innovate and start companies, or simply to change jobs. And job loss would be less devastating.

The concept of healthcare being a right is not new. It was embedded in 1948 in the fundamental international framework, the United Nations Universal Declaration of Human Rights, which asserts that healthcare should be accessible to all citizens, and it has been included in the framework for many countries as they've developed their healthcare systems. Here it is, as written in Article 25 of the declaration, the drafting of which was led by former First Lady Eleanor Roosevelt:

> Everyone has the right to a standard of living adequate for the health and well-being of himself and of his family, including food, clothing, housing *and medical care* and necessary social services, and the right to security in the event of unemployment, sickness, disability, widowhood, old age or other lack of livelihood in circumstances beyond his control.[9] (Emphasis mine.)

When I first started learning about social justice, I was drawn to the American political and ethical philosopher John Rawls and his "veil of ignorance" concept. In short, Rawls argues that in order to ensure a just society, citizens must make choices from an original position of equality and ignorance, without knowing what gender, race, abilities, tastes, wealth, or position in society they will have. Put another way, he challenges us to ask ourselves what kind of society we would create if we didn't know what our gender, race, or socioeconomic status would be at birth.

For me, healthcare is an integral part of a just society. As Rawls describes it:

> *Medical care*, as with primary goods generally, is to meet the needs and requirements of citizens as free and equal. Such care falls under the means necessary to underwrite fair *equality of opportunity* and our capacity to take advantage of our basic rights and liberties, and thus be normal and fully cooperating members of society over a complete life.[10] (Emphasis mine.)

This is particularly true for a democracy. A democracy depends on fully participating citizens, and in order to be fully participating, those citizens' basic needs must be met. For example, since 1870, all states in the US have had tax-subsidized elementary schools, consistent with the belief that universal public education is vital to an informed, participatory citizenry. Why not consider healthcare the same way? Citizens need to be healthy to be fully participating members of our society.[11]

As President Obama concluded in 2010, "In the wealthiest nation on earth, no one should go broke because they get sick. In the United States of America, *health care is not a privilege for the fortunate few—it is a right.*"[12] (Emphasis mine.)

Most Americans agree. There are, in fact, decades of survey results indicating that Americans support the notion that healthcare is a right. Moreover, the results from a 2017 poll suggest the country may be shifting even further toward supporting the expansion of healthcare access, with 63 percent saying it's the federal government's responsibility to make sure that all Americans have healthcare coverage.[13] Women are slightly more likely to believe this (65 percent of women versus 60 percent of men).

Over the past fifty years, we've actually been taking incremental steps toward establishing healthcare as a right. First, we covered the elderly and disabled with Medicare, then most of the poor with Medicaid. Next, we required emergency rooms to take all comers. Then, for people without health insurance coverage through their jobs, we required insurers to cover preexisting conditions and offered some subsidies to make that coverage more affordable—thanks to the ACA. This focus on protecting people with preexisting conditions has brought us much closer to treating healthcare as a right in the US.

Americans are supporting those steps, little by little. Since 2010, researchers have been polling Americans to gauge support for the ACA. Interestingly, the results show that the ACA is viewed more favorably since the repeal efforts in 2017, indicating that Americans support, and are willing to defend, the expansion of Medicaid, consumer protections, and other ACA provisions when they perceive them as being under threat. As part of this, there has been a major shift in awareness and thinking about preexisting conditions and what it means to protect them. Here again, women tend to show stronger support, believing that it should be illegal to deny coverage for preexisting conditions.[14]

So, if most of us agree that it's the federal government's responsibility to make sure that all Americans have healthcare coverage, and if the ACA moved the country in that direction, why were so many politicians trying to dismantle it in 2017? That year, the individual mandate penalty—so essential to the fabric of the ACA—was repealed. The Congressional Budget Office projects that thirteen million will lose coverage by 2027 due to these changes.[15] Since then, other protections granted under the ACA have been undermined, and the entirety of the law is threatened.

Why do we seem to be taking this big step backward—and more importantly, what can we do to support key provisions of the ACA and keep moving toward healthcare for all? How can women take the lead? I'll begin answering those questions by reviewing how our healthcare system evolved to become the patchwork of coverage it is today.

CHAPTER 2

■ ■ ■ ■ ■ ■

HOW WE GOT HERE AND WHERE WE STAND

After 100 years of trying, finally, we passed health care for all Americans as a right for all, not just a privilege for a few. It honored the vows of our founders, of ... healthier life, liberty, the freedom to pursue our own happiness."

SPEAKER NANCY PELOSI, on the passage of the Affordable Care Act[1]

I'LL NEVER FORGET March 22, 2010, the day I returned from a week "off the grid" in Central America. As I exited the plane at Miami International Airport, I glimpsed the front page of the *Miami Herald* and read the headline in big, bold letters: "Healthcare History." My heart sank. Did this mean the push for health reform was over? Throughout that winter, Congress had been debating the Affordable Care Act. Knowing how polarized the issue had become, I assumed the worst—that the legislation had failed.

But then I took a closer look.

Underneath the headline was a photo of Speaker Nancy Pelosi, beaming, gavel in hand, and surrounded by smiling colleagues. That's when I realized that the seemingly impossible had happened—the Affordable Care Act had passed. Indeed, "healthcare history" had been made, and the US was on its way to making healthcare more accessible for millions of Americans.

Why was this such an unforgettable, historic event? And even more fundamentally, why is government involved in our healthcare, anyway? Let me take a step back and explain why health reform is so political and then turn to how our country's patchwork quilt of healthcare coverage evolved.

Healthcare access has always been political. It's part of the ongoing debate in our country over the role of government, as epitomized by the current positions of the Republican and Democratic parties. The ever-present tension around the extent of government's role in our lives comes into play particularly when the free market fails to meet the needs of its citizens. Healthcare presents just such a challenge because the free market will supply healthcare only to those who can *afford* it. It doesn't automatically allocate healthcare to those who *need* it. This makes healthcare a privilege rather than a right in the US. To address this inequity, government has to get involved. And with that involvement comes politics.

A HISTORY OF PATCHWORK COVERAGE

When our country was founded back in 1776 and for most of its first one hundred years, there was no formal healthcare system. But during the past one hundred years or so, as medical science developed new treatment options and healthcare grew into a national system, people wanted access to the new options, be they hospital treatments or drug therapies. To pay for these expensive new treatments, they needed a coverage solution. Over time, patches of coverage have been created and stitched into place. As you'll see, the process has often started with a call for universal healthcare coverage—only to end with a political compromise that meant settling for something less, a patch.[2]

Teddy Roosevelt led the first charge for universal healthcare coverage in 1912 when he ran for president as the candidate of the Bull Moose Party, formally known as the Progressive Party. Teddy was defeated, but the universal coverage idea did not die. In 1934, his distant cousin, Franklin D. Roosevelt, created the Committee on Economic Security, chaired by labor secretary Frances Perkins, the first woman to serve in a US cabinet. Part of the committee's charge was to find ways to expand social insurance, including health insurance, and its work led to the passage of a landmark law, the Social Security Act of 1935, which established the Social Security and welfare programs. The committee was unable to reach a compromise on the issue of health insurance (due to strong opposition from organized medicine—doctors were concerned about the government interfering with both the doctor-patient relationship and their fees)[3] so nothing more was done about healthcare in Roosevelt's New Deal era.

Enter Harry Truman, who became president after Roosevelt's death in 1945. Truman is credited with being "the president who was the strongest advocate for comprehensive, compulsory health insurance,"[4] and in 1945 he proposed the Fair Deal program, which included a bill for universal coverage. It, too, faced strong opposition from the American Medical Association and never came up for a vote in Congress, as the nation turned its attention to other pressing issues, including the Cold War. Truman later called his failure to pass universal healthcare "the greatest regret of his life."[5]

The US took the path of least resistance while other countries, including Britain, were making more concerted efforts to ensure equal access to healthcare for all their citizens. Many established the foundations of their universal healthcare systems after World War II, in concert with the United Nation's 1948 Declaration of Human Rights, which included medical care as a basic human right. (More on this in chapter 9.)

Outside of the government arena, private health insurance solutions were also developing back in the 1930s, first to cover hospital stays, and then to cover physician services. Employers started to offer these health plans, bit by bit, encouraged by hospitals that were looking for ways to cover patient costs when their revenues declined during the Great Depression. The number of Americans with some form of health insurance grew to twenty million by 1940, which was about 9 percent of the population at the time.[6]

This number grew tremendously during World War II. Labor was in short supply and the US government had implemented wage and price controls. Importantly, they excluded health insurance from these controls. So, to attract labor, more companies began to offer health insurance as an employee benefit. Almost two-thirds of working Americans had health insurance coverage for hospital stays by 1950.[7] This number continued to grow thanks to the enactment of another key benefit by the federal government: excluding health insurance benefits from payroll taxes.[8] (This tax exclusion is now a huge benefit, worth at least $250 billion per year, and it accrues primarily to middle- and upper-class people.)[9]

By the mid-1950s, healthcare was back on the agenda as Americans realized that relying on employer-sponsored insurance for the nation's healthcare solution left out an important, and sympathetic, group: the elderly. Activists, including organized labor, pushed hard for Medicare. It took many attempts, but they overcame opposition from doctors and insurers, and in 1965 the Social Security Amendments established the Medicare program, thanks to the efforts of many and the leadership of President Lyndon Johnson, who sought to achieve some of President John F. Kennedy's goals after he was assassinated. Medicare covers people who are sixty-five years and older, or disabled, regardless of income, and it is funded by a combination of payroll and general taxes, plus premium payments.

The Medicaid program was also established as part of the Social Security Amendments of 1965. Another important patch in the coverage quilt,

Medicaid began by covering only very low-income people in specific catego-ries (typically mothers and children, not childless adults). It has expanded over the years. Combined, Medicare and Medicaid extended healthcare coverage to thirty-four million Americans within the first five years of the programs, and they now serve well over a hundred million people.

Whereas Medicare is entirely located in the federal system, Medicaid was established as a joint federal/state program. It's important to remember the differences between the two systems because this has implications for where political pressure should be directed. Back in 1965, states were given the option to implement the Medicaid program or not. They were provided with federal money to do so, but they had to come up with "state matching funds." It took eighteen years for every state to join the program; Arizona was last, in 1983. This dynamic of widely varying approaches to Medic-aid continues to the present day, as states consider whether to expand their Medicaid programs to cover more people.

Establishing Medicare and Medicaid were major achievements, but the push for even more comprehensive coverage continued. Richard Nixon proposed an expansion of the employer-based health insurance system, in-cluding a requirement for employers to offer health insurance, stating that "no American family should be denied access to adequate medical care be-cause of an inability to pay."[10] At the time, his approach was rejected by leading Democrats, who wanted a Canadian-style single-payer government program; when Nixon resigned in August 1974 because of the Watergate scandal, his initiative lost all momentum.

The next major push for national health reform happened in 1993, spon-sored by President Bill Clinton and led by his wife, Hillary Rodham Clin-ton. They proposed a market-based, consumer-friendly plan, rather than a universal, mandatory government program originally favored by Demo-crats. This resulted in only lukewarm support from some Democrats and advocates. The Clintons' plan retained a role for private insurers and gave people seeking insurance coverage choices, plus subsidies if their employer didn't offer coverage. In an interesting bit of foreshadowing, Republicans responded with a counterproposal that included a mandate for people to buy health insurance. Neither proposal was able to gain much popular support, and the Clintons' proposal was staunchly opposed by the insurance industry, which was able to pour millions of dollars into a public ad campaign against the prospective legislation. Thanks to this negative publicity blitz, the gen-eral public—always wary of government's involvement in their healthcare decisions—began to fear that they wouldn't be able to keep the insurance they had.[11]

Although the Clinton proposal ultimately failed, it set a precedent for Democrats to focus on market-based solutions moving forward. It also led the way toward an incremental, bipartisan win in 1997: the Children's Health Insurance Program (CHIP), which expanded Medicaid-like coverage to eight million children in lower-middle-income families.

Coverage expansion continued under the next president, George W. Bush, this time with a focus on Medicare. President Bush, a self-proclaimed "compassionate conservative," secured the biggest expansion of the Medicare program since inception: the addition of an outpatient prescription drug benefit (Medicare Part D). The establishment of Medicare Part D was another significant incremental win in the march toward universal coverage. It strengthened the coverage quilt by stitching in an additional patch where patients had previously been required to pay for all of their own prescription drug coverage.

THE NEED FOR THE ACA

Incremental expansions of Medicaid and Medicare still left a tremendous number of people without health coverage (forty-five million in 2009), and that number was expected to grow significantly (to between fifty-four and sixty-one million) by 2019.[12] By the time Barack Obama was elected president in 2008, the coverage quilt was becoming bare in even more places. The employer-based healthcare system was eroding, and the Medicaid program was stuck in the zone of covering only the neediest, with enormous variation in coverage from state to state. For those who lost their employer coverage, there were not many good alternatives in the individual market. Insurers were concerned that people would game the system by not purchasing health insurance until they got sick, an economic concept called "adverse selection." So insurers would charge more for, or just plain exclude, people with preexisting conditions who they knew would likely cost them money. As a result, the insurance being sold in the individual market in most states was unavailable or prohibitively expensive if you had a preexisting condition, and cheap if you didn't, and it didn't cover much in most cases.

The resulting situation was bad for everybody. People with serious illnesses could not find insurance to cover themselves, and many either lost all of their savings and went bankrupt or didn't receive care.

Lots of people (myself included) felt like the healthcare system was failing the sick in a big way. While insurance companies claimed their practices were developed to protect those who opted for coverage without waiting for a medical need from those who were trying to "game the system," many people couldn't find insurance for a host of legitimate reasons—maybe they moved, or switched jobs, or got divorced, or maybe they'd had a condition since birth. Those affected by preexisting condition exclusions were in a painful minority, and it was difficult for them to band together and get traction politically with their issues.

One of the most unconscionable reasons for a preexisting condition–based exclusion was domestic abuse. This exclusion was legal in eight states and Washington, DC. The practice trapped women in physically abusive relationships. If they left an abusive husband and were no longer covered under their husband's health plan, they couldn't get a new health plan. Why? Because being abused counted as a preexisting condition for which they could be denied coverage.[13]

Back then, another one of the most egregious insurance practices in the individual insurance market was known as "rescission," which was a retroactive cancellation of a health insurance policyholder's coverage. One day you think you have coverage, and the next day you don't—and that happens to be the day you really need it. When the House Committee on Energy and Commerce conducted an investigation into the practice, it found that it was widespread in insurance companies, and that bonus structures often incentivized employees to review claims "with an eye toward rescission in every case in which a policyholder submits a claim relating to leukemia, breast cancer or any of a list of 1,400 serious or costly medical conditions."[14] Tens of thousands of policies were rescinded due to alleged failure to disclose a health condition entirely unrelated to the policyholder's current medical problem or failure to disclose a medical condition that a doctor had never told someone about, and due to innocent mistakes by policyholders in their applications (which were extremely complex and confusing), as well as failure to disclose the medical condition of one family member.

Victims of rescission testified before the investigating congressional subcommittee and their stories are deeply troubling. A woman named Robin Beaton shared her story. She went to a dermatologist for acne, and her dermatologist used a word meaning "precancerous" in her chart. The next month, she was diagnosed with invasive HER-2 genetic breast cancer, a very aggressive form of cancer that required an immediate double mastectomy. The week before her surgery, her insurer called her and told her that her chart was red-flagged because of a word the dermatologist used that they interpreted as meaning "precancerous" and they would not pay for her surgery. Her dermatologist called the insurance company to explain that he didn't actually mean precancerous but was only describing her acne, but they refused to reinstate her policy. Robin was in an incredibly precarious situation: her hospital wanted a $30,000 deposit, but she didn't have enough to cover it for a surgery she needed immediately. It wasn't until she called her congressman to put pressure on her insurer that the insurer relented.[15] Many weren't as lucky as she was and died as a result of their coverage rescission.

I'm not trying to paint insurance companies as villains. Especially before enactment of the ACA, the problem was that in the absence of market rules, they were in a competitive race to pay out fewer claims—if they failed at this race, they could be priced out of the market and potentially go out of business. Given these harmful practices, and the large and growing number of uninsured people, a solution was needed.

This was an opportunity for a universal coverage solution, but a "fill-the-gap" solution was chosen instead. Universal coverage was a bridge too far, in part because of lessons learned from the Clintons' attempt at health reform in the 1990s. And there was the benefit of having a working solution already in place at the state level: Massachusetts had a "fill-the-gap" model that balanced liberal and conservative philosophies and closed the growing gap between employer-based coverage and Medicaid. This model had achieved near-universal coverage in the state, so it had the potential to fill a big gap nationally. This working model (which I'll describe in chapter 5) became the foundation of the ACA of 2010.

POLITICS AND THE ACA

Healthcare reform was a signature issue in the 2008 presidential election campaign: Voters demanded that the candidates address it. Front-runner Hillary Clinton was an acknowledged expert on the issue, given her previous work during her husband's presidency. The other front-runner, Barack Obama, also indicated his commitment to the issue, releasing his health reform plan as a campaign document in May 2007. As the election drew closer, congressional leaders began preparing for Democratic victories—they and their staffs had rolled up their sleeves and begun drafting a health reform plan.[16] Notably, Senator Ted Kennedy provided a tremendous amount of leadership on this issue before his death.

The 2008 election was a major victory for Democrats. Barack Obama won the presidency with the largest share of the popular vote obtained by a Democrat since Lyndon Johnson was elected in 1964 (which was key to enacting Medicare and Medicaid one year later). The House and Senate also had Democratic majorities, which in the Senate was large enough to be filibuster-proof. With this level of strong electoral support, the Democrats moved quickly on health reform. Many of the participants in the process were veterans of the failed attempt at health reform under the Clinton administration. They knew they had to move fast, before the political tide turned. They also knew that they needed to start with something that was already working—Congress doesn't like to enact things that are dramatically new.

They benefited from the strong support of the new president: Barack Obama proved time and again that health reform was one of his top priorities, despite the significant pushback he got, even from his own staff. Some of the Democratic leaders in Congress worked hard to find bipartisan support for the ACA, to no avail.[17] Even some Democrats wavered in their conviction through this grueling process. It took fierce leadership and constant pressure from outside groups such as Planned Parenthood to keep the new legislation on course—especially when it came to women's health issues.

The Speaker of the House, Nancy Pelosi, is an unsung hero in this effort—she kept her party together, even through a contentious debate on abortion coverage. A mother of five and a strong supporter of addressing women's health issues, Pelosi ensured passage of an ACA that covered abortions and remedied long-standing injustices for women. As Cecile Richards, the former head of Planned Parenthood, later wrote, "Nancy didn't blink."[18]

The passage of the ACA was possible in large part because of the Democratic majority in the House and Senate. But pressure campaigns from outside groups also played an important role in keeping legislators focused—especially when it came to women's health issues. It's important to remember that we as citizens can make a difference even after elections by holding our representatives accountable for the promises they made.

A̲T THE TIME, proponents of the ACA hailed the legislation not only as a way to expand healthcare access but also as an unprecedented boost to

America's economy and entrepreneurial spirit. Speaker Pelosi summed it up from the floor of the US House of Representatives:

> I believe that this legislation will unleash tremendous entrepreneurial power into our economy. Imagine a society and an economy where a person could change jobs without losing health insurance, where they could be self-employed or start a small business. Imagine an economy where people could follow their passions and their talent without having to worry that their children would not have health insurance, that if they had a child with dia-betes who was bipolar or [a] pre-existing medical condition in their family, that they would be job-locked. Under this bill, their entrepreneurial spirit will be unleashed.[19]

Vice President Joe Biden was even more succinct. "This is a big f*ing deal," he said.[20]

By contrast, detractors saw the ACA as a "centralized health dictator-ship"[21] or an "ambitious power grab"[22] that "will cost the federal government untold billions."[23] Upset about this perceived overreach by Democrats, Re-publicans began attempting to repeal the ACA as soon as it was enacted. Court challenges were brought, filed the day after the ACA was signed into law. President Obama vetoed the one repeal bill that made it to his desk and he (mostly) prevailed in court. But after Obama's two terms in office, this firewall was replaced by a Republican president and a Republican-majority Congress.

Republican candidates campaigned on repealing the ACA throughout the 2016 presidential election. When Donald Trump won, he promised to repeal the ACA on "day one." Shortly after Trump took office in 2017, he set about making good on his campaign promise to repeal and replace the ACA, with Republican majorities in the House and Senate willing to oblige. Once it came down to the details, though, he found that redesigning the US healthcare system was harder than he thought. "Nobody knew health care could be so complicated," he admitted on live television.[24]

Undeterred, Trump and the Republican leadership set forth a series of bills they hoped would do away with "Obamacare" once and for all. These bills included provisions like removing protections for people with preexist-ing conditions and limiting Medicaid spending by "block granting," or cap-ping the amount of federal funding for states. However, Trump and the GOP leadership ran into public opinion roadblocks when people found out that the ACA's consumer protections would be eliminated, and when the Congressional Budget Office (CBO) determined that the bills would cause twenty-four million to thirty-two million Americans to become uninsured.[25] Polls showed that support for the ACA grew as the "repeal the ACA" efforts persisted.[26] Republicans faced fierce opposition from their own constituents, who increasingly turned to activism: from rallies to packed town hall meetings, many of which went viral on social media, there was unrelenting public pressure to save the ACA. Republicans also got strong pushback from states: a bipartisan group of governors lobbied hard against the Medicaid block-granting ideas, and encouraged bipartisan solutions.[27]

In the end, Congressional Republicans were divided about how to proceed: some wanted to repeal the ACA outright, and others only wanted to repeal it if they could replace it at the same time. The repeal and replace bills were ultimately defeated or withdrawn, culminating in a dramatic "thumbs down" deciding vote by the late senator John McCain, Republican of Arizona.

As a result, the ACA remains law, but Trump has used executive actions to undermine it, upsetting the law's delicate balance. Republicans were also able to claim a partial victory with the repeal of the individual mandate penalty at the end of 2017. (As noted earlier, the individual mandate was first called for by Republicans in the 1990s and was implemented at the state level by Republican governor Mitt Romney in Massachusetts in 2006. Ironically, the ACA penalty was repealed by a Republican Congress and Trump as part of the Tax Cuts and Jobs Act in 2017.) Millions will lose coverage due to this change.

THE MARKET ONLY TAKES US SO FAR

One of the biggest reasons why health reform attempts have been so political is that many Americans idealize the free market and resist government involvement while others see it differently—this leads to an inevitable clash. Let's dig into this a bit.

Throughout my career, I have heard that our country's healthcare woes would be solved if we just let the free market "do its job." That would mean letting supply and demand, a.k.a. the "invisible hand" of the marketplace, determine who gets access to healthcare, and how much healthcare they can have.

There are many problems with this notion. First, the separation of who's paying for healthcare (insurers) from who's consuming it interferes with the supply and demand mechanism. If consumers don't know the full price of their healthcare and don't have to pay for it directly, they are less sensitive to prices and may "overconsume." For example, they may request extra office visits or tests (such as MRIs) even if unnecessary. And consumers won't shop around for the best deal if they aren't bearing the cost. As a result of this lack of connection to price, healthcare providers can charge high prices to insurers while being protected from the drop in consumer demand that would happen in a traditional marketplace. (This is an important underlying reason why healthcare is so expensive, and insurance premiums are so high.)

Another dimension of this issue is that consumers who can't afford insurance coverage are shut out of the market almost completely, especially if they have healthcare needs. This is related to the skewed distribution of risk pool incentives, whereby sicker people want coverage while insurers want to keep their costs down, so they'd prefer to avoid high-cost enrollees. Before the ACA, the individual insurance market was designed this way—it was most expensive and least accessible to the sickest people. Unfortunately, a healthcare system organized purely on free-market principles will be deeply skewed toward inequality—especially since markets in the US are organized to maximize investors' income. (I would like to see them be more concerned with stakeholders, not just shareholders, as called for in the principles of "conscious capitalism.")

The market model for healthcare coverage also fosters constant churning, instead of long-term doctor-patient relationships. Plus, it requires informed consumers, which is a problem, given low rates of financial literacy and other challenges.

And then there are the other "market failures" economists see, such as consumers having imperfect information, suppliers (like some insurers and hospitals) having monopoly power, and externalities (these are the "spillover effects" that market prices don't take into account, and they can be positive or negative). Since these market failures, by definition, can't be solved through the market alone, they require government intervention.

The upshot: when it comes to healthcare, there are significant limits to what a free market can achieve. The free market can determine how much of a good should be produced, and at what price, to bring the most value to those who produce and consume that good. What the market *cannot* do is produce goods that are both universally needed and more expensive than many can afford. So, a pure free-market system will never be able to provide universal healthcare coverage—in fact, it can't even get close. The power of the consumer to walk away is what causes products to reach an equilibrium of price and product supplied. To walk away from the sale of a house or movie ticket is one thing. To walk away from a mammogram appointment or an insulin shot because of high price is not merely the free market finding equilibrium; that act can incur tremendous damage on individual health, families, and society.

In the case of healthcare, the free market doesn't work. It fails spectacularly, allocating healthcare only to those who can afford it, not those who need it. As a result, some have called for "extensive government intervention," because it is "more likely to result in the achievement of societal objectives than are market forces supplemented by minimal government intervention."[28] We can debate how much is the right amount, but the bottom line is that government intervention is needed. And that means the solution to our healthcare crisis must be political.

T HE US IS NOT UNIQUE in having to wrestle with how to provide healthcare to its citizens. The issues of market failures, lack of affordability, and the need for government involvement exist in other countries as well. But other countries have gone further in solving the problem. I believe strongly in looking beyond our borders to see what we can learn. We need to, because our patchwork approach to health coverage leaves us bare in too many places, unlike all of the other developed countries that have all achieved universal coverage.

The US is getting a terrible return on its healthcare spending investment, and if we want to maintain our position as a world leader, we need to address it. The US spends about twice as much per person on healthcare as other developed countries, yet has worse health outcomes than other developed countries. In fact, the US has a higher mortality rate, a higher rate of deaths amenable to healthcare, a higher disease burden, and more hospital admissions for preventable disease.[29] This is outrageous, given that the US is spending well over $3 trillion on healthcare each year. How can we accept such a low return on investment?

Don't get me wrong—I love to feel proud of America. But I don't feel proud when I look at how our healthcare system compares to those of other countries.

■   ■   ■

IN SUM, THERE have been many attempts to enact universal healthcare coverage in the US over the past seventy years, and they have resulted in incremental progress. Several attempts have been bipartisan, some of which have been successful. Viewed through a universal coverage lens, however, they are only partial successes: each has added or expanded a patch on the coverage quilt. Yet each fell short of establishing a right to healthcare in the US.

The US has relied on the marketplace to provide most of its health insurance coverage for the country, and this fundamental choice has led to the patchwork approach. But it's clear that the market cannot provide a solution to universal healthcare on its own—there are too many market failures. The need for government involvement means that we must find and embrace a political solution. As I'll explain in the next chapter, women have led change in the healthcare system in the past and can lead the way toward universal coverage now.

It's time to make healthcare a right.

■ ■ ■ ■ ■ ■

CHAPTER 3

WHY WOMEN CAN BE THE DRIVERS OF UNIVERSAL HEALTHCARE

The most common way people give up their power
is by thinking they don't have any.

—ALICE WALKER, author of *The Color Purple*[1]

EARLY IN THE MORNING on January 21, 2017, I stood at the corner of Independence Avenue and Maryland Avenue SW. Not far from the US Capitol building, shoulder to shoulder in a sea of other protesters, I waited for the Women's March on Washington to begin. I saw people holding handmade signs that read "I will not go quietly back into the 1950s" and "Well-behaved women seldom made history." Others were starting to chant refrains such as "This is what democracy looks like!" There with my mother, my oldest daughter, my sister-in-law, and my friends, I sensed the awakening of a community spanning generations and all walks of life. At that point, though, I had no idea that this event would turn out to be the largest single-day protest in American history, with up to five million of us advocating for issues like women's rights, immigration reform, the environment, and tolerance.

But the Women's March wasn't only massive; it was also high-energy, determined, and peaceful. And the combination of these elements was what made that day so incredibly uplifting and empowering. The 2017 March inspired countless women to engage in efforts to promote equality and justice, whether by getting more information, voting, joining committees, or even running for public office. It was one of the key factors from that year that inspired me to write this book.

In short, the collective action of the Women's March created positive change and showed us once again that activism works. Activism has proven itself over the course of many years and many issues, including healthcare, where in 2017, organized resistance defeated numerous attempts by Republican legislators to repeal the ACA. The threat of millions of people losing health coverage was real, and Americans across the country responded with activism: marching, protesting at town hall meetings, flooding Congress with calls. I participated in many of these events and was continually astounded by not only the turnout, but the energy, determination, and focus that I witnessed.

And through it all, women have been leading the way. Women were at the forefront of the public protests and made the vast majority (86 percent) of calls to Congress defending the ACA.[2] More recently, in the 2018 midterm elections, women reported voting for Democrats over Republicans (59 percent to 40 percent),[3] presumably due in part to the importance of the healthcare issue in that election, and Democrats' consistent stance of protecting access to healthcare.

But if we want our government to recognize healthcare as a right, women need to do even more. A primary reason is to address the challenges women face as caregivers—the healthcare system is not meeting our needs.

The ACA expanded healthcare coverage to twenty million Americans, established consumer protections, and made healthcare affordable for many. But it didn't go far enough. Too many people still lack health insurance coverage, and too many others are worried about not being able to afford theirs. To put it in terms I've used before, we need a fleece blanket that provides full coverage, not a patchwork quilt with bare spots. However, the healthcare system isn't going to ensure access by itself. We, the people, must make it happen. How? With political activism.

As I explained in chapter 2, we need government involvement to ensure a competitive marketplace and guarantee access to coverage. Based on other successful activist movements, it is also clear that a key catalyst to government action is meaningful cultural change. That's why it's critical to work on these two issues in tandem: if we drive the culture change to *expect* healthcare for all, then the legislators should follow.

Women have successfully driven cultural and political change in the past—on a massive scale through the women's suffrage movement, and in more targeted efforts to ensure that women's health issues were recognized and treated fairly by the medical establishment. But women's potential to drive the movement for universal healthcare is as yet unrealized, as many of us aren't sure how to join the fight. Women are an untapped resource of leadership, voices, donations, and, very importantly, votes.

In terms of leadership potential, women remain grossly underrepresented in positions of power, including in elected offices and high-level corporate positions. Specifically, women make up only 24 percent of members of Congress, 6 percent of Fortune 500 CEOs, and less than 14 percent of experts interviewed on Sunday TV talk shows.[4] The statistics are worse for women of color (they make up just 9 percent of Congress while representing fully 35 percent of the population). These numbers show where women's increased participation can transform the leadership landscape—and the sooner, the better. Even with the recent gains in the 2018 midterm elections, at the rate we are going, it will take more than fifty years before women are 50 percent of Congress. I doubt I will live to see the day, unless we demand that society pick up the pace.

But elevating more women to leadership positions is only part of the solution. Unfortunately, too many of us fall into the trap of thinking that we can't make a difference unless we are rich and powerful or hold a senior-level position. This ignores the power of collective action, which can take on many forms, including exertion of economic power through our purchases, investments, and donations.

For example, men donate more to political organizations than women do. In fact, donations from men account for two-thirds of all political donations.[5] This gives men more access and influence in the political process, which is where systemic issues are addressed. Women, by contrast, donate more to nonprofit organizations—which is great, but donations to charities do not translate into advocacy or legal changes, which means our donations don't address the systemic issues.

This is where we as women must get out of our comfort zones. Traditionally, many women have focused their time and energy on volunteering for smaller local activities, typically centered on fundraising. While that can be a choice that feels comfortable and perhaps avoids controversy, it can also take time away from addressing bigger budget items and the systemic issues. As one of my favorite bumper stickers reads: "It will be a great day when our schools have all the money they need, and our air force has to have a bake sale to buy a bomber."[6]

HARNESSING THE POWER OF COLLECTIVE ACTION

When Americans are asked to identify where collective action has been most powerful, they often think of the civil rights movement of the 1950s and 1960s, which culminated in the Civil Rights Act of 1964 and the Voting

Rights Act of 1965. Earlier in our history, there were other powerful movements, including those led by abolitionists who fought to end slavery and
suffragists who fought for women's right to vote. As a child, I was inspired
by the farmworkers movement, crystallized by the grape boycott, which
brought attention to inhumane working conditions for Latinos. At the same
time, the women's movement of the 1960s and 1970s increased opportunities for women, improving access to better-paying jobs and educational opportunities[7] and establishing reproductive rights. These movements raised
awareness, changed hearts and minds, put pressure on those in power, and
ultimately impacted laws.

There has not yet been a massive social movement in support of universal healthcare. Instead, the social movements for healthcare have been more
grassroots and piecemeal, organized by groups, such as the women's health
movement and AIDS activist groups, focused on specific causes. They are
often led by patients, based on their experiences. (This contrasts with "elite
health reform," which has relied more on research and professional expertise.)[8] The patient groups advocate for their own healthcare issues initially;
some, like ACT UP and the National Council for Senior Citizens, advocated for universal healthcare later. ACT UP leaders realized that universal
healthcare was the only way to ensure different patient groups weren't pitted
against one another in a battle for coverage. There have also been organizations created that support grassroots activism for expanded healthcare coverage, such as Families USA and Community Catalyst, as well as numerous
state-based organizations, but none have (yet) set off a national movement
for universal healthcare.

Through it all, women have found ways to make changes in healthcare
by leading from where they are: from early calls for universal coverage, to
changes in the provision of healthcare services, women have a long tradition
of standing up for what they need and believe in. Women's health journalist Barbara Seaman noted that "American women have been the 'perennial
health care reformers.'"[9] Now, women are standing up for their rights once
again, galvanized by the aftermath of the 2016 election. Capitalizing on this
energy provides a tremendous opportunity to push for universal healthcare.

A BRIEF HISTORY OF WOMEN'S HEALTH ACTIVISM

Women's activism in our nation has deep historical roots, even if it wasn't
featured prominently in our history books. And it started with a focus on
health at its most basic level: survival. Some brave women acted individually:

one of the earliest examples was Mumbet, an enslaved woman in Massachusetts. Terribly abused by the man who owned her, she sought her freedom in court—and won, aided by a lawyer who took her case. The precedent established by Mumbet's case helped lead to the abolition of slavery in Massachusetts in 1783 when the court determined that slavery was inconsistent with the state's constitution.[10]

Other brave women joined forces and worked together: Female factory workers protested against working conditions in the Lowell mills in Massachusetts and catalyzed a nationwide labor movement in the 1830s—this contributed to the establishment of much-needed workplace safety regulations.

Decades later, as the labor movement picked up steam in the early 1900s, activists rallied for more support. The American Association for Labor Legislation proposed a "compulsory health insurance" plan that would cover workers' costs when they were ill (it was modeled on programs that were already happening in England and Germany). Women involved in the trade union and suffrage movements supported the proposal in part because it included maternity benefits for women workers. They rallied and demonstrated during a massive march on the state capitol in New York in 1919.[11] The proposal passed in the state senate but died in the state's House of Representatives. Ultimately, even though the legislation failed, it planted seeds for future attempts at health reform.

During this time, Frances Perkins, who would later become the first woman appointed to a federal cabinet position, witnessed the 1911 Triangle Shirtwaist Factory fire in New York City, which killed 145 people.[12] A social reformer who was working as a professor of sociology at Adelphi College, Perkins was prompted by the event to alter her career path so she could address labor issues. She went on to hold several government leadership posts in New York as an industrial commissioner. As President Franklin D. Roosevelt's only secretary of labor, Perkins's crowning achievements were passage of the Social Security Act and the Fair Labor Standards Act, which broke new ground in American social welfare policy and brought major improvements to the welfare of all Americans. The Social Security Act also provided the foundation for Medicare and Medicaid (though it would take three more decades to get there).

At the local level, women in the labor movement took the lead in establishing a health center for garment workers who struggled with tuberculosis and other health problems. The International Ladies' Garment Workers' Union (ILGWU) created and staffed such a clinic in 1913. Pauline Newman led the clinic for over fifty years. Seeing that the needs of her patients and the community extended far beyond what the ILGWU was able to handle in their clinic, she became an early champion of universal healthcare. As she said, "The great mass of workers are not in any position to look after their own problems. That is why [the ILGWU] is in favor of health insurance and social insurance. We can take care of ourselves, but who are we? A mere hundred and fifty thousand."[13] She continued to advocate for universal coverage for the rest of her life.

Meanwhile, also in 1913, a group of wealthy women in New York City began a crusade to fight cancer. Their group became the genesis of the American Cancer Society. The women, who were socialites and philanthropists as well as members of the Women's Municipal League, pushed a group of doctors to launch a campaign to "educate the public to recognize the early symptoms of the disease," similar to what had been done for tuberculosis. The *New York Times* headline read, "Rich Women Begin a War on Cancer." The campaign was focused on educating women, because the activists had noticed that women had twice the cancer rates that men did. They wanted to replace the fear and denial of a cancer diagnosis with a "message of hope and early detection."[14]

The women's suffrage movement coincided with a variety of other women-led social initiatives, including the temperance movement and efforts to address immigrants' needs. The work, which included the establishment of settlement houses, focused on improving the health and well-being of the population. Women's activism at the local level built toward making change at the national level: scholars have traced the connection between women's social welfare work during the Progressive Era in the 1890s to 1920s and their attempts to influence public policy in Franklin Roosevelt's New Deal era of the 1930s.

Black women were also working to address healthcare issues at the same time that white women were leading these early reforms, as chronicled by feminist historian and professor of women's studies Susan L. Smith in her book *Sick and Tired of Being Sick and Tired: Black Women's Health Activism in America, 1890–1950*. Black women, however, had the added challenge of living in a legally segregated society where they were completely disenfranchised.[15] But that didn't stop them.

In the 1960s, civil rights leader Fannie Lou Hamer declared that she and all black people were "sick and tired of being sick and tired." This strong sentiment developed well before the civil rights era: Smith notes that there has been a "continuous, unbroken line of black women's health activism since at least the 1890s."[16] Black women were leading and supporting health improvement initiatives for decades, long before there was any formal healthcare movement.

But black women activists had to pressure the health system for change from outside the system itself. The medical profession was so segregated that there were very few professional opportunities for black people, and especially for black women. As a result, laypeople—especially midwives—played a key role in bringing attention to public health. Black women recognized that "health [w]as indissolubly linked to the poverty and other socioeconomic factors that hindered black progress."[17] They were strongly aware of what we now call the social determinants of health, since they lived them.

Indeed, there were huge disparities in health outcomes for black and white Americans. These became more measurable following the Civil War, as state boards of health were being established in the South. For example, the death rate of the black population in New Orleans was reported to be four times that of the white population following the 1878 epidemic of yellow fever. Rather than recognizing the systemic roots of this issue, however, white Southerners in the post–Civil War era tended to blame black people for their health problems, believing they were racially inferior. Black leaders saw it very differently: after attending a 1906 conference on black health in Atlanta, W. E. B. Du Bois concluded that the difference in mortality seemed to be explained by the "conditions of life."[18] In saying this, he drew attention to the outrageousness of the claims of black inferiority and pointed to environmental and social solutions. These systemic solutions, like improving sanitation, were already being used in the North to combat the spread of communicable diseases.

In the face of such strong societal barriers, black women from all walks of life led health improvement activities and provided support at the community level through their roles as midwives, mothers, and public health nurses. Middle-class black women used their connections with sororities and churches to raise funds and provide needed staff and supplies to black hospitals, including Provident Hospital and Nurses Training School in Chicago. The Alpha Kappa Alpha (AKA) sorority created the AKA Mississippi Health Project, which set up mobile health clinics every summer during the Great Depression. These and other efforts paved the way for future participation in national health reform efforts.

As more and more black people migrated out of the South, their overall health became a national issue, not just a Southern one. Black middle-class activists tried to get their communities included in public policy through awareness-raising campaigns like National Negro Health Week. They succeeded in getting the Office of Negro Health Work established in 1932, as one of President Franklin D. Roosevelt's New Deal programs. The office supported black health education and funded black healthcare workers' grassroots efforts to improve health in their communities. It also hired black doctors to expand Negro Health Week programs. (The office's work was discontinued in 1950 as needs changed and integration efforts got under way.)[19]

Securing this national attention was key to unlocking federal funds for establishing community health centers and other initiatives. This led to the creation of the Delta Health Center in Mound Bayou, Mississippi, an all-black community in the Delta region. It was one of the first two community health centers established in the US (the other was in Boston), and the first rural community health center. Cofounded in 1965 by a team of black and white civil rights activists, the Delta Health Center was modeled on a clinic one of the founders had seen in a Zulu tribal reserve during a trip to South Africa in the 1950s.

The Delta Health Center founders believed that healthcare is a right. They also believed that the community should be able to shape their healthcare solutions, so the founders guaranteed them a role in the design and control of their health services. Dr. Helen Burnes, a black ob-gyn, joined the center in 1968, and many local black women were trained as nurses and nurse's aides; by 1969, twenty-one of twenty-six nursing staff were longtime local residents.[20] Lula C. Dorsey, born to sharecroppers, joined the center as a community health organizer, and received further training while working there. Thanks to the center's community empowerment model, Dorsey was able to obtain her GED and later a PhD. She came back to serve as the center's executive director.[21]

From their lived experience, the black women at the Delta Health Center knew that the center needed to focus on more than medical care; it needed to address the environmental conditions—also called the social determinants—that were affecting the health of their community. They insisted on serving those broader needs through health education, job training and placement, childcare, and even a farm cooperative to raise healthy food. Feminist scholar Jennifer Nelson summed it up this way: "Through their involvement, local black women ensured that the Delta Health Center

conformed to values about health and healthcare held by the black community—not those imposed by white medical practitioners on blacks."[22]

This provided a stark contrast with how blacks were treated by the
healthcare system in the rest of the South and elsewhere. As Nelson explains, "African American women in Mound Bayou, Mississippi, shaped
healthcare to suit their community and individual needs by becoming cen-
trally involved in the creation and maintenance of a community health center that served them."[23]

The Delta Health Center provides an excellent example of how to use
healthcare as a point of entry for social change. In fact, it paved the way for
many other health clinics, all of which contributed to the spread of the idea of
universal access to healthcare. Black women worked at the community level
in health centers and elsewhere, laying the groundwork for later generations
with greater social power to have a more direct influence on public policy.

These historical highlights demonstrate both the power and the limits
of community efforts not backed by the strength of national public health
policy to address people's health needs. As historian Susan L. Smith put it,
"Current calls for the transformation of the healthcare system are not new;
they are deeply rooted in the history of African-American health reform,
which demonstrated the necessity of universal health provisions."[24]

THE WOMEN'S HEALTH MOVEMENT

In conjunction with the Second Wave of feminism in the 1960s and 1970s, a
women's health movement was born. There were many issues ripe for attention, due in part to the sexist bias of the medical profession (in those days,
over 90 percent of doctors, including ob-gyns, were men).[25] These issues
included the overmedicalization of the birthing process and the prevalence
of unnecessary surgical interventions, including hysterectomies, Cesarean
sections, and radical mastectomies.[26] The movement focused on women being able to make their own decisions about their bodies. But it also sowed
seeds for broader health reform, as women called attention to the fact that
all women needed to be able to access quality, affordable healthcare.

It started with health education. The groundbreaking book *Our Bodies,
Ourselves* and its author organization, The Boston Women's Health Book
Collective, sprung out of a conference workshop called "Women and Their
Bodies." Attendees gathered to share information, only to realize that they
had more questions than answers. A year and a half later, they self-published
Our Bodies, Ourselves, which later became a best seller. It was viewed as radical

in many areas and banned in some. But it was oh-so empowering. (I got my first copy from a college friend as a bridal shower gift in 1990, and I still remember its graphic content and how much it taught me about women's health.) In 2012, it was named by the Library of Congress as one of the most influential books in terms of shaping American culture.[27]

Soon, a variety of advocacy groups convened. They were small initially: there were almost two thousand self-help women's medical projects between 1969 and 1975. Many of these grassroots advocacy organizations were composed of women who had participated in civil rights, antiwar, and student movements of the 1960s. These grew into national organizations: first, the National Women's Health Network, then the National Black Women's Health Project. The national organizations worked to increase awareness of women's health issues, including, for example, the laws governing them, and to "act as a counter-force to organized medicine and the drug industry."[28] They advocated for more research and funding of women's health issues, including breast cancer. They were joined in activism around women's issues generally by other national organizations, such as the YWCA, the National Council of Negro Women, the Older Women's League, and the Children's Defense Fund.

By the 1980s, the women's health movement had gone beyond the grassroots level. There were an increasing number of "professional advocates," including doctors, scientists, lawyers, and corporate executives.[29] At this point, women were sufficiently established as professionals in the workforce that they could bring a feminist lens to healthcare institutions by serving as health educators, lobbyists, and service providers.

At the same time, black women continued to embrace and promote healthcare as a tool for community development and individual empowerment as they became active in the reproductive rights and the black women's health movements in the 1970s and 1980s.[30] The Black Women's Health Imperative is one organization that brought multiple approaches together, including individual and systemic, working at the grassroots and national levels. Founded in 1983, the organization focuses on health equity and social justice for black women. It has tackled health reform through advocacy and public policy, health education, research, and leadership development. A strong supporter of the Affordable Care Act, the Black Women's Health Imperative continues to fight against ACA repeal. It has also worked on identifying and addressing health disparities (which were really not discussed by policymakers until the 1970s women's health movement). Its leaders take a holistic and grassroots approach by also supporting community clinics and self-help. Their work is based on an empowerment model: women shouldn't have to struggle alone—they can reduce stress by identifying their challenges and obtaining the resources to make change.[31]

One of the big successes of the women's health movement was restoration of control of the birthing process to women. Childbirth had become overmedicalized, to the point where women were sedated or forced to give birth in positions that were more convenient for the doctor than the mother. Now women have choices in where and how they have their babies—from delivering with midwives at home to giving birth at full-service hospitals—and more insurance options to help them pay for this care.

A major portion of the women's health movement has been focused on reproductive rights. Women have fought long and hard for the right to determine their pregnancies. From gaining access to birth control to being able to have an abortion safely and legally, the battles continue to the present day and consume a tremendous amount of time and energy.

Reproductive rights activists have often been at the forefront of calling for universal healthcare. There are many examples, including the Puerto Rican activists who protested the death of a woman who received a legal abortion in a New York City hospital in 1970 and linked her death to her poor-quality healthcare.[32] Planned Parenthood threw its weight behind getting the ACA passed in 2010. As Cecile Richards, the former CEO of Planned Parenthood, said at the time,

> The Affordable Care Act represents the biggest advance for women's health in 45 years. . . . Millions more women will be covered. Women will no longer be charged more for care than men. And women will not be denied coverage because they are sick or pregnant.[33]

No one's healthcare is truly a right until everyone has access to good, affordable healthcare. Planned Parenthood's support of the ACA draws attention to the way a lack of health coverage prevents other rights—including access to safe and legal abortions—from being upheld in our nation, and highlights the ways women are disproportionately impacted.

Perhaps one of the greatest successes of the women's health movement was the outlawing of insurer practices that penalized women simply for being women. Insurers used to charge women more for individual market health insurance, and many excluded maternity coverage; in fact, 80 percent of individual market policies excluded maternity coverage in the 1970s.[34] The ACA outlawed all of this in 2010 and went even further: it requires no co-pay for birth control and preventive screening exams.

In sum, while the women's health movement may be better known for its powerful critique of the sexism of the medical profession, there has also been an undercurrent of the need to make healthcare a right. In 1971, the first edition of *Our Bodies, Ourselves* pointed out that women without access to healthcare were dying of *preventable* cancers, such as cervical and uterine. Decades ago, the authors wrote, "We believe that *health care is a human right* and that a society should provide free health care for itself" (emphasis mine). Women today need to keep pushing for the rights we've long known should be ours.

L OOKING BACK AT THIS HISTORY, it is clear that many women were able to overcome enormous obstacles in pursuit of their activist agendas. Yet there were many more who didn't become activists, because they faced obstacles that were too difficult to overcome—obstacles that range from the systemic to the personal. Some, such as discrimination, have both elements: they have systemic roots which are then internalized at a personal level. Whatever the source, obstacles can hold women back from fully participating in a social movement.

When obstacles become internalized, the psychological barriers to activism deepen. These psychological barriers include insecurity and discomfort with controversy. Women experience more self-doubt than men, due in part to the ways in which we are socialized from an early age to second-guess ourselves and downplay our achievements.[35] This is exacerbated by the negative stereotypes of women as activists: we are perceived as "strident" or "militant." Feminist activists have often been demonized in this way.

Moreover, women are frequently punished for any emotional display, especially when we're angry. Feminist journalist Rebecca Traister has documented the many ways in which women are treated as an oppressed majority in the US. Her writing dials in on how women's anger has long been discouraged in our culture "via silencing, erasure, and repression."[36] Many cultures view women's anger as evidence of a lack of self-control, so that any woman who expresses her anger is easily dismissed as crazy, irrational, bitter, or even hysterical. Feminist Andrea Dworkin, known for her unabashed challenge to patriarchy in the 1970s, nailed it when she talked about the threat of violence, verbal or physical, against women leading women to "lower our voices. Women whisper. Women apologize. Women shut up. Women trivialize what we know. Women shrink. Women pull back."[37] Even women who do speak up often end up trying to stabilize an escalating situation by downplaying their own passion, rather than risk being seen as dangerous or crazy.

Unfortunately, these obstacles are not merely historical—they are present today, and they can still be difficult to overcome. And yet, as feminist poet Audre Lorde said, "Every woman has a well-stocked arsenal of anger . . . focused with precision, it can become a powerful source of energy, serving progress and change."[38] Moreover, there is power in our numbers, and our numbers are growing: we are beginning to realize that "we are not as isolated in our rage as we had been led to believe."[39]

There are plenty of things to be angry about. Lack of universal healthcare is one of them. Imagine the power that women would have to make social change if we didn't let these obstacles get in our way and truly banded together, rising up in fury. This potential power is left unrealized if we let ourselves be divided. Traister points to reporting around the Women's Marches, with headlines that focused on the divisions between the women, rather than the power of what united them. She suggests that journalism is biased since it is (still) controlled by the white male establishment. This means that a strong, united group of women could be threatening to that establishment. It is certainly an example of where culture change is needed, regarding who controls the stories and the narrative in our media sources.

Throughout history, anger has been at the root of all social change. Traister reminds us that when women suppress their emotions, especially anger, we surrender much of our potential power.[40] So if we are going to tackle our healthcare coverage problems, we need to figure out how to harness our anger and channel it toward the cause of making healthcare a right. That said, we have to be aware that not all anger is treated the same: "Black women's fury is treated differently from white women's rage; poor women's frustrations are heard differently from the ire of the wealthy."[41]

To overcome this, we need to realize our collective power and form alliances across women's groups, like the Women's Marches did. The Women's Marches strove to be inclusive and intersectional: the marchers addressed racism, misogyny, healthcare, the environment, and much more. Many white women who participated in the Women's Marches were newly awakened to these feelings of rage. Many men participated and witnessed this rage. One-third of the marchers had never been to a political protest before.

And the first Women's March was the largest single-day protest in US history. The marches were followed by massive amounts of political organizing, which was in turn followed by record numbers of women running for office. One significant result: in the 2018 midterm elections, women picked up a historic number of seats in Congress. In the words of Dolores Huerta, longtime feminist and farmworker activist, "Sí, se puede!" (Yes, we can!)

WOMEN HAVE PROVEN THEMSELVES capable of strong and persistent activism on health (and many other) issues, locally and nationally. We have built awareness and overcome obstacles, both personal and systemic. We now need to bring it all together, holistically and impactfully, with a movement for universal healthcare.

Historically, any major attempts at universal healthcare have come from the top, driven more by policy wonks than by grassroots activists. Today, however, there's a growing consensus in the US that the lack of affordable, guaranteed healthcare coverage is a problem, in part because the ACA gave us a more tangible taste of the promise of affordable universal coverage. And it brought the spotlight to healthcare in a big way. But for all that the ACA solved, it also came up short. Millions of people are still uninsured or are worrying about losing the coverage they do have. The concern has been loud and clear, broadcast on posters I saw throughout the Women's March— and have continued to see ever since: Keep Your Hands Off My Healthcare. United We March. Keep America Covered. Healthcare Is a Human Right. And so many more. We need to convey these messages so that we can rally more people to the cause and get a consensus on the need to act.

Looking ahead to new "targets of opportunity" for feminists and the women's health movement, universal healthcare should be high on our list. In addition to our challenges as caregivers, women are more vulnerable to gaps in the employer-sponsored insurance system and cutbacks in Medicaid. In the next three chapters, I'll explain how and why the current healthcare coverage system comes up short, especially for women.

CHAPTER 4

EMPLOYER-SPONSORED INSURANCE WON'T SAVE US

The workplace is being globalized, digitized and roboticized at a speed, scope and scale that we've never seen before.

—THOMAS FRIEDMAN, *Thank You for Being Late*[1]

I REMEMBER WHEN I got my first full-time job after college, working to raise money for the YWCA. I was so excited to tell my parents about what I'd be doing, but my mother cut me off almost immediately.

"Does the job have health insurance?" she asked.

"Yes," I answered, a bit dumbfounded. Why was that her first question? I didn't have enough life experience at that point to understand my mother's concern. But I learned. My employer-sponsored plan was there for me when I was rear-ended by another driver when I was twenty-two years old (an accident that resulted in an emergency room visit and a neck brace). It was there to help cover my birth control pill prescription, and there to cover prenatal care and delivery of my three babies, including a somewhat risky twin pregnancy. At every stage of my life, my employer-sponsored plans have been there for me, making healthcare affordable.

Fast forward to today and employer-sponsored insurance remains commonplace, covering almost half of Americans. That said, it is far from the rock-solid benefit we once counted on. Employers are continually redefining what they can afford or want to offer, which means that this patch is stitched together with significant variation throughout, contributing to the overall "crazy" nature of our national coverage quilt. On top of that, most job-based plans are shrinking in value as employees are required to contribute more, through hikes in premiums, deductibles, and other out-of-pocket spending.

And yet, most who have health insurance through their jobs are reasonably happy with it: Surveys show that anywhere from half to three-quarters of people with employer-sponsored insurance are satisfied with their coverage, although the number appears to be declining.[2] For one thing, people with job-based plans tend to have access to a broader array of healthcare providers than others do. But how have women fared in a health insurance system so deeply rooted in employer-based coverage? Do job-based plans meet their needs?

WOMEN AND EMPLOYER-SPONSORED INSURANCE

The share of women in the labor force has grown significantly since the 1960s, from 40 percent in 1966 (the year I was born and the year that IBM's company policy required my mother to leave her job because she was pregnant) to 57 percent now.[3]

But women in the workforce are a little less likely to be eligible for employer-sponsored insurance coverage through their own jobs than are men. In addition, men are more likely to take up this coverage.[4] The ability to cover family members makes up for this difference: an estimated 25 percent of working-age women are insured as dependents of their spouses.[5] So, in the end, women are just as likely as men to be covered by employer-sponsored insurance one way or another.

Even so, since women are more likely to be dependent on a spouse for health insurance coverage, women can be at a distinct disadvantage if they divorce. Indeed, divorce leaves some sixty-five thousand women uninsured each year.[6] These are women who are not participating in the labor force or who work part time, or who are in jobs without employer-sponsored insurance.

And even women who have their own employer-sponsored insurance are often disadvantaged: Not only do they earn less pay than men, but a recent review of employer benefits revealed that companies employing a majority of women offered less generous health coverage than those employing a majority of men.[7] This ties in with the fact that female-dominated jobs (which are predominantly in healthcare and service industries) are less well-compensated than traditionally male jobs, like manufacturing.

Moreover, women are adversely affected by the limited availability of employer-sponsored insurance for the part-time and low-wage jobs they often "choose" due to family or personal obligations. Survey data shows that women are more likely to be responsible for eldercare than men and spend more time caring for children as well.[8] As journalist Natalie Shure explains, "The strains of childrearing and elder care make women more likely to seek more flexible employment, like part-time, remote, or freelance work. These forms of employment tend not only to pay less, but are less likely to include health insurance benefits."[9]

Approximately 25 percent of employed women work part-time, compared to only 12 percent of men. Put another way, women comprise almost two-thirds of part-time workers.[10] But part-time workers are far less likely to be offered health insurance: only 42 percent were offered coverage in 2015, compared to 85 percent of full-time workers.[11] They are also less likely to be offered other benefits, such as paid sick leave or family leave, as shown in the figure below. This can be a tremendous burden for single mothers who need both family coverage and more time in their day for childrearing. Women of color are especially impacted, since they hold the majority of jobs at or around minimum wage.[12] (See figure 4.1.)

FIGURE 4.1 Part-Time Workers and Low-Income Women Are Less Likely to Be Offered "Fringe Benefits" by Their Employers

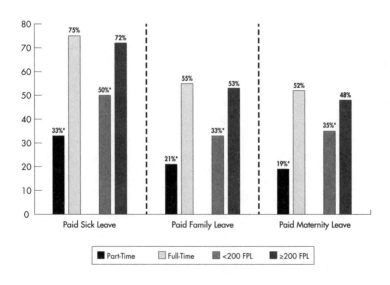

Source: Kaiser Family Foundation, *Kaiser Women's Health Survey*, 2017.

Note: Among women ages 18–64 employed full- or part-time. The Federal Poverty Level (FPL) was $20,420 for a family of three in 2017.

*Indicates a statistically significant difference from full-time and ≥ 200% FPL; p < .05

This strain of caregiving and employer-sponsored insurance limitations is compounded for women by several other factors. For instance, many women find themselves in the impossible predicament of having to choose between caring for a loved one or working outside the home, simply to remain eligible for employer-sponsored insurance.[13] During urgent health episodes, like childbirth or a relative's long illness, many women leave their jobs or have to take unpaid time off to provide care and comfort. According to the US Department of Labor, nearly one-third of women who take unpaid time off for their own or a dependent's health issues fall into serious credit card debt.[14]

Finally, women are impacted by another limitation of employer-sponsored insurance plans: the availability of birth control. Although the ACA requires health plans and self-insured employers to cover birth control for free, employers who are religious or have moral objections have been exempted from this requirement because of litigation that reached the US Supreme Court. The Trump administration tried to widen this exemption in late 2017, making it easier for any company to claim a moral objection and exclude birth control from coverage.[15] Although this rule was blocked in federal court,[16] employer-sponsored insurance plans for large companies have fewer requirements and protections under the law than individual and small group plans, and can be susceptible to the erosion of benefits.

A BRIEF HISTORY OF EMPLOYER-SPONSORED INSURANCE

Given how detrimental employer-sponsored health insurance can be to women and children, how did it become the dominant form of health insurance in the United States? It happened unintentionally. No law created it, nor was there any grand plan by a politician, a trade group, or an industry player. Rather, the employer-based system that supports one-third of the spending in the $3.65 trillion healthcare industry evolved as a by-product of economic circumstances, laws that were intended to address other issues, and changes to the US tax code.

The American employer-sponsored insurance system was born in the late 1920s when a smart administrator from Baylor Hospital in Dallas decided that the purchasing habits of cosmetics consumers would translate well into healthcare. It was an era of significant medical breakthroughs, including penicillin, vaccines, and epidural anesthesia. However, increasingly sophisticated hospitals had high cost structures and struggled to generate enough revenue to cover these advances. People had a hard time paying for large hospital bills but would "spend a dollar or so at a time for cosmetics and not notice the high cost."[17] If a large number of people were to spend small sums of money over a long period of time, this would enable the average consumer to pay for a large hospital bill, and simultaneously provide a consistent stream of revenue for the hospital. Baylor Hospital struck a deal with a group of public school teachers in the area, who each paid fifty cents per month in exchange for the promise of twenty-one days of free care at the hospital should any of them become ill.

This payment model quickly proliferated across the country. Hospitals liked it because of the appeal of consistent revenue, and it was the only way consumers could afford healthcare during the Great Depression. These same principles hold true today (although nobody has called a healthcare premium a "small sum of money" in a very long time).

A few years later, when the United States joined World War II, the federal government imposed controls on wages and prices so that the wartime labor shortage wouldn't translate to a high cost for consumers. This policy inadvertently led to an explosion of fringe benefits that were not subject to wage controls (like pensions, paid holidays, vacations, and health insurance), which companies used to attract employees. Then, in 1943, the Internal Revenue Service (IRS) gave employer-sponsored insurance an additional boost by making it tax-free; the policy was made into law by Congress in 1953, the first year of the Eisenhower administration. Today, employer-sponsored insurance is the biggest and fastest growing exemption in the US tax code—to the tune of over $250 billion a year.

This tax exemption is a primary reason why employer-sponsored insurance evolved into the dominant form of health insurance in the United States. Healthcare premiums are tax-deductible for employers, and employees don't pay income taxes on premiums. This is a substantial benefit for employers and employees alike. That said, it only helps those who work for employers who can afford to pay for health benefits. And the more generous the benefit, the bigger the tax exemption, so people with higher incomes benefit more from the tax exemption. In fact, the upper- and middle-class benefit tremendously from this deduction, often without being aware of the benefit. This exemption is considered to be "regressive" tax policy—benefiting the wealthy more than the nonwealthy—as opposed to "progressive," which raises an important issue of fairness. (Stay tuned for more on this in chapter 11, where I discuss ways to fund universal healthcare.)

The shift in tax policy stimulated the adoption of employer-sponsored insurance. It covered just 9 percent of the population in 1940 but by 1953 had grown to 63 percent of the population. Today, that percentage is down to 49 percent, but employer-sponsored insurance remains an appealing form of worker compensation for many: when employer-sponsored insurance is offered, most eligible employees—76 percent, or 84 million people—accept it. (This coverage extends to almost twice that number of people—157 million—when the employees' dependents are taken into account.) After all, the average employee only has to pay 18 percent of their premium for individual coverage (or 31 percent for family coverage), and their employer pays the rest. However, this "take-up rate" has eroded in the past decade for reasons I'll explore below.[18]

PROBLEMS WITH EMPLOYER-SPONSORED INSURANCE

Despite the relative popularity of employer-sponsored insurance, Americans can't rely on it to solve our healthcare coverage crisis. That's because the availability of employer-sponsored insurance is shrinking, and those who have it are receiving fewer benefits than before. In fact, as I'll explain in chapter 6, 25 percent of people with employer-sponsored insurance are now considered to be "underinsured." In addition, as I've already shown, women tend to be disadvantaged in their access to job-based plans. And perhaps most problematic of all, the current megatrends don't favor employer-sponsored insurance.

Megatrends are global and sustained forces that have long-term impacts on societies. For example, globalization and the acceleration of technology are megatrends that are shifting our economic reality in profound ways. The flow of knowledge worldwide is virtually unstoppable, leading to new work arrangements that require flexibility and autonomy.

In short, globalization is opening up numerous economic opportunities for individuals and companies both within and beyond our borders and it is forcing companies to be nimble. As a result, workforce needs are constantly shifting, and that means employees often get dislocated. Without safety nets that transcend the boundaries of jobs, people will increasingly face "health coverage insecurity" related to potential job loss. Jobs were already becoming far less permanent than they were when my father had his career at IBM, over thirty years ago. And when the Great Recession hit in 2008, millions of people lost their jobs (close to one in six workers).[19] This huge job loss hit people at all income levels, as entire companies and jobs disappeared. Newspapers were filled with stories about Lehman Brothers going under and General Motors making cuts (including discontinuing the Pontiac and Saturn lines), and the 170,000 small businesses that closed. Some people found new jobs, but it took a while, and the new jobs were not necessarily as good as the old jobs in terms of benefits.[20]

Millennials were deeply affected by this experience, as they watched their parents suffer. They paid close attention during the recession and its aftermath and have since been less prone to taking financial risks, such as taking on mortgages and credit card debt, or starting their own businesses.[21] Millennials also support the general concept of a larger government which provides more services and a safety net to ensure a minimum quality of life. According to a Pew Research survey, 57 percent of millennials would prefer a bigger government providing more services, compared to 50 percent of Gen Xers, 43 percent of baby boomers, and 30 percent of the "silent generation." Support for universal healthcare shows an even stronger effect: 67 percent of millennials believe it is the federal government's responsibility to make sure all Americans have healthcare coverage, compared to 52–58 percent of the other age groups.[22]

A major by-product of the Great Recession as well as the globalization and technology megatrends is the advent of the "gig economy," in which companies offer short-term contracts to freelancers who in turn trade benefits like health insurance for flexibility. Jobs in the gig economy rarely offer health insurance—in fact, it is estimated that anywhere from 15 percent to 37 percent of gig workers are uninsured.[23] According to the Bureau of Labor Statistics, which tracks the work categories that make up the gig economy, about 10 percent of the US workforce, or fifteen million people, participated in "alternative work arrangements," such as freelance and temp positions, as their main job in 2017. Six million people considered themselves to be "contingent workers," meaning they were working on temporary projects as their main job. (Contingent workers and those in alternative work arrangements are counted separately and numbers can overlap.)[24]

The gig economy structure is expanding globally, and some sectors, like transportation (think Uber and Lyft), are growing more dramatically than others. Despite the hoopla about the gig economy, however, the share of workers whose main job is in a gig category has actually gone down slightly since 2005, even with the prevalence of Uber and other disruptive innovators. For most, gig work brings in extra cash—it is not their primary source of income.

However, many industry watchers predict these numbers will increase again, which could mean that what's happened with transportation could ripple to other sectors. Freelance work like computer coding, copywriting, and virtual assistance is increasingly made possible by new technology, and many employers predict that they will shift more of their workforce to non-permanent status.[25] "We are seeing a convergence of cost reduction initiatives and the need for employers to have more agility, with workers looking for more flexibility. Together, these objectives are driving a shift toward a contingent workforce," says Tony Steadman, a top leader from the global financial firm Ernst & Young who advises companies on human capital issues.[26] More contingent jobs means fewer jobs with health insurance. Or, as one freelancing humorist put it: "Our health plan is: Don't get sick."[27]

An interesting side note: a series of lawsuits in recent years have questioned whether platform operators like Uber should be considered employers. If they are, their employees would receive benefits like unemployment insurance, workers' compensation, and time off. As of this writing, this issue is still being debated in the court system, although it seems that the "not employees" side is likely to win out, and gig economy participants will not be entitled to protections bestowed by the Fair Labor Standards Act and many other workplace laws. If more people move into the gig economy, the country will face important questions about how to protect these workers in times of health crises.

On the flip side, for those workers who have job-based plans, a major limitation is that the plans don't travel from job to job. Switching to a new job typically means a change in insurance plan, a change in doctors, and a disruption in care—hassles that some economists say cause job lock among American workers.[28] This phenomenon, in which employees who remain in a position only for the benefits, harms the overall economy because it stifles entrepreneurship and innovation and keeps people working at jobs that may not match their skills. As economist Brigitte Madrian noted, "The productivity of the economy as a whole will suffer if individuals who would like to move to more productive jobs are constrained to keep their current positions simply to maintain their health insurance."[29]

For those workers who lose their employer-sponsored insurance when their job situation changes, they can keep their health plan for eighteen months (through a benefit called COBRA),[30] but it will take a big bite out of their wallet. Many people in this situation now opt to buy a cheaper health insurance plan through the exchanges that were established by the ACA—more on that in chapter 5.

In addition to all of this, the employer-sponsored insurance system is under tremendous stress from the rising cost of healthcare, which dwarfs the growth in the rest of the economy. Between 1999 and 2017, the US economy grew a respectable 42 percent.[31] But over that same time frame, employers' health insurance premiums grew a whopping 300 percent (for both individual and family coverage).[32] The powerful economic force of high healthcare costs has affected employer-sponsored plan designs in various ways, but the common theme is that employers are trying to reduce their costs.

Of course, the most obvious way for an employer to do that is to simply stop offering employer-sponsored insurance. Indeed, over the past two decades, there has been a gradual decline in the share of employers who are offering health insurance, from 68 percent down to 57 percent.[33] This has been driven mostly by the share of small firms (those with fewer than fifty workers) that are not offering health insurance. Like individual market purchasers, small employers don't have as many insurance companies knocking down their doors trying to get their business, and they typically don't have the negotiating power that larger firms do (although recent federal rules may open the door to small employers grouping together and purchasing large group plans).[34]

Larger firms, particularly those with more than a hundred employees, have mostly maintained their commitment to offering coverage. This phenomenon can be partially attributed to the ACA requirement for large employers to provide health insurance or be subject to a penalty. However, large employers are also better able to handle the increasing cost of health insurance because they can negotiate good rates or opt for a cheaper self-pay contract. Their negotiated plans are also subject to fewer rules and regulations and are generally cheaper than those sold to small employers. That said, some large employers have pulled back on how much they are paying for coverage to spouses and dependents of employees.

The upshot: people, such as my children's preschool teacher, who work for small firms or nonprofits are less and less likely to have healthcare coverage.

Another way that employers are addressing rising healthcare costs is by shifting expenses to employees. From 2005 to 2018, the amount workers pay toward health insurance premiums increased at a greater rate than that of employer contributions (51 percent versus 30 percent). In 2018, the share of premium contributions paid by covered workers averaged 18 percent for single coverage and 29 percent for family coverage. While these percentages have remained somewhat stable since 1999, the amount paid monthly has increased significantly, especially for family coverage, due to the rising cost of healthcare. The average monthly premium contribution paid by workers for family coverage has more than doubled: it went from $222 per month in 1999 to $462 a month in 2018 (adjusted for inflation).[35]

In addition to employees having to contribute more toward premiums, employers are asking their employees to contribute more toward out-of-pocket costs (known as cost-sharing, like co-pays and deductibles). That's because employee cost-sharing helps to reduce the employers' costs and helps to keep healthcare spending down by reducing the utilization of healthcare—in other words, by motivating employees to go to the doctor less or to limit their use of medications. This was demonstrated in the 1970s with the RAND Health Insurance Experiment, which found that people with no cost-sharing tended to consume more healthcare than those with cost-sharing. The most notable (and troubling) finding of the study was that people with cost-sharing reduced their utilization of both unnecessary and necessary care equally.[36]

Deductibles, in particular, are becoming an increasingly common form of cost-sharing.[37] Deductibles make policyholders responsible for the entire amount of their healthcare bills up to a certain point, so they may find themselves wondering, "Do I really need that visit to the specialist?" The answer tends to change if you ask people with a $40 co-pay versus people who may be short of their deductible, leaving them responsible for paying a specialist's entire $2,000 bill.

High-deductible health plans (HDHPs) are an increasingly popular form of employer-sponsored insurance because they keep costs down for employers and seem cheap for employees—but they're only cheap for healthy people. To help pay deductibles, many HDHPs allow people to save money tax-free in a health savings account (HSA) that can be used only for healthcare purchases. The problem is that these HDHP plan designs are so difficult to comprehend that only one in five policyholders understands that preventive office visits, medical tests, and screenings are exempt from the deductible.[38] As a result, many forgo preventive care.[39] But again, it's not just preventive care that ends up by the wayside; as mentioned, the RAND health experiment showed us that people faced with cost-sharing reduce both necessary and unnecessary care equally.

Clearly, from a kitchen-table economics perspective, people are being forced to put Band-Aids on a very broken situation—that's all they can afford. As paycheck growth has stagnated, rising healthcare costs are taking a bigger bite out of take-home pay. On top of this, over half of American workers face a deductible of more than $1,000, yet more than half of Americans can't cover a $1,000 unexpected expense.[40]

For all the reasons described above, there is tremendous variation in how employers offer insurance, and employees can have a hard time finding a plan that meets their needs. Beyond the cost-sharing issues, there are other variables, such as who and what is covered, and where care is available. Some employer plans cover only employees; others offer health benefits for spouses and dependents of employees, though that may be at an additional expense to the employee.[41] Some firms offer health plans that allow policyholders to see almost any doctor or go to any hospital; others limit the choice through "narrow networks." And then there are the extras, like dental and vision insurance, which some firms offer, and others don't. Some employer-sponsored insurance plans for mid- to large-size companies don't cover essential health benefits—the ACA does not require them to.[42]

Why is there so much variation in employer-sponsored plans? In general, companies have different levels of resources and commitment to covering employee benefits. As a result, it makes a big difference whether you are employed by a small company or a large one. Large companies tend to have more resources to devote to employee benefits, including health insurance. It also matters if you are in an industry competing for talent (like high tech) or one that might treat you more like a commodity (like retail or hospitality). If you are in a highly competitive industry, odds are that your employer wants to keep you happy so that you stay in your job. Similarly, if you are in a labor union, you are most likely enjoying a robust benefit package that has been negotiated with your employer. And finally, the leadership philosophy of the company you work for, and its generosity toward employees, matters a great deal—some leaders are more willing to "share the wealth" than others.

One of the strengths of employer-sponsored insurance is that employers can work with insurers to help innovate new approaches to health coverage that allow employers' healthcare dollars to stretch further, while also promoting high-quality outcomes. A few pioneering employers are engaging with "centers of excellence," programs with extremely high levels of expertise in a particular area or procedure, and can provide care at large scale with low cost and reliable output.

Exploring ways to get to universal healthcare shouldn't automatically mean dismissing the employer-sponsored insurance system that's already in place, because that could disrupt and upset millions of people. It would be very challenging to implement such a massive change. As we look to universal healthcare options, we'll want to leverage the strengths of the employer-sponsored insurance system even as we attempt to move away from some of the challenges that come along with it.

I T BOILS DOWN TO THIS: the availability and value of employer-sponsored insurance is eroding due to the megatrends of globalization and technology, as well as related market forces. As things currently stand, women are less likely to benefit from employer-sponsored insurance and are more at risk of losing it. Even though women are the chief medical officers of their households, they are personally powerless in the face of these realities. Ultimately, we need health coverage that transcends corporate shifts and job loss, and employer-based health insurance won't get us there.

Despite these problems, many employees are happy with their employer-sponsored insurance coverage—for the moment, that is. Industry groups, including labor unions, lobby to protect employer-sponsored insurance, or at least to keep government from overregulating it. And an industry of benefits advisors has grown up around this private system. So even though many corporate CFOs would be happy to take the health insurance expense off of their books, or at least rein in its higher-than-inflation rate of growth, employer-sponsored insurance is an established benefit in most mid- to large-size companies, and it is likely to stay.

Addressing the shortcomings of employer-sponsored insurance to provide adequate health security for all workers will require a bigger systemic and compassionate solution—one that must be based on making healthcare a right. The ACA was a step in that direction; let's take a closer look.

■ ■ ■ ■ ■ ■

CHAPTER 5

THE ACA ONLY
GOT US PARTWAY

Today we have the opportunity to complete the great unfinished business of our society and pass health insurance reform for all Americans. That is a right and not a privilege.

—NANCY PELOSI, speech before Affordable
Care Act vote, March 2010[1]

WHEN THE AFFORDABLE CARE ACT passed in 2010, over forty-five million Americans were uninsured—most were working but didn't have health insurance through their own or a family member's job. The ACA dramatically improved their health insurance coverage opportunities, but it didn't just appear out of thin air. It was based on a model that I helped to implement in Massachusetts four years earlier.

Massachusetts passed its groundbreaking health reform law in 2006, and the bill was signed into law in Boston's historic Faneuil Hall amidst great fanfare. At the time, I was across the river, working at Harvard University, but news traveled quickly. Many of my former colleagues were there, and they told me that everyone in the room, including Governor Mitt Romney, a Republican, and Senator Ted Kennedy, a Democrat, was buzzing with optimism. The law was developed with bipartisan input and had the support of healthcare advocates, government officials, and business leaders. It established the Massachusetts Health Connector, the first state-run health insurance exchange in the US. A few years later, once it was clear that the Health Connector was solving the problems it was designed to solve, both the Massachusetts state health reform law and the Health Connector went on to serve as models for the ACA.

■ ■ ■

S HORTLY AFTER THE CEREMONY in Faneuil Hall, I was hired as the founding deputy director of the Massachusetts Health Connector. My job was
to put a team together to build this first-ever public marketplace for private
health insurance. For me, a policy wonk, the opportunity to help implement
the new law was my dream job. States are "laboratories of democracy," and
this was my big chance to implement a health reform program that I deeply
believed in, one that would open up coverage to people like my children's
preschool teacher and so many more. I poured my heart and soul into it.
The whole team did.

Before the establishment of the Massachusetts Health Connector, the
state—like the rest of the country—had a growing number of uninsured
people, most of whom were working. The individual insurance market was
expensive, and the threat of losing federal funding for the uninsured people
who used "free care" (also known as "uncompensated care") in our hospitals
was real.

At the Health Connector, our primary goal was to achieve "near-
universal coverage." We didn't dare say *universal* coverage, because we were
doing something that had never been tried before in the US, and we didn't
want to be perceived as overreaching. I certainly knew from my previous experiences with implementing government programs that there were plenty
of things that could go wrong. Our secondary goal was to make the individual health insurance marketplace more affordable for those who were
buying insurance on their own.

When I first took the job, I hoped that the health reforms we were in-
stituting might be replicated in other states, but success was a long shot. We
had an aggressive launch timeline, unproven program ideas, and technologi-
cal challenges, plus we feared that people would reject the individual mandate—any one of these risks, if realized, could turn public opinion against
us before we achieved any wins. Luckily, thanks to a phenomenal team that
brought diverse experience, dedication, and grit, along with external stakeholders who stayed committed to health reform's success and supported us
through challenging times, we were able to exceed expectations. With the
whole country watching, Massachusetts developed a new system for accessing healthcare that could work for the nation.

THE INDIVIDUAL MARKET IN MASSACHUSETTS

As its name implies, individual insurance, also known as "nongroup insurance," is bought by individual people instead of by a group of people (like

a company or a union). It's the patch on the national coverage quilt that covers about 6 percent of Americans: people whose jobs do not offer health benefits (such as independent contractors and self-employed people) or who are unemployed and don't qualify for public programs such as Medicare or Medicaid. The most common reason why people purchase health insurance through the individual market is to protect them from financial risk—75 percent of survey respondents indicated this was the case. This was followed by "for peace of mind" (66 percent) and "you or a family member has a health condition that requires ongoing medical care" (41 percent).[2]

Prior to the ACA, the individual insurance market was riddled with complexity and inconsistencies. In most states, you couldn't buy the insurance if you were sick, or if you could, it was outrageously expensive. It was affordable only if you were completely healthy. This left large numbers of people without a viable coverage option if they didn't have employer-sponsored insurance. Massachusetts had a slightly different problem—we had an even higher cost of individual insurance because, unlike most other states at the time, Massachusetts had a law that guaranteed the opportunity to buy coverage to everyone, even if they had poor health. Unfortunately, this meant that many sick people were buying insurance, and using their insurance for costly care, and the insurers had to charge accordingly, with higher premiums. Other states excluded sick people from the individual insurance market and could therefore charge lower premiums to healthy people. So, one of the primary goals of Massachusetts health reform was to lower the cost of insurance in the individual market while still guaranteeing coverage to sick people. Another goal was to bring similar benefits to the small group market.

To accomplish this, Massachusetts initiated its health reform law and built in several policy innovations, including an individual mandate that required nearly every resident to sign up for health insurance.[3] The law provided free health insurance to low-income residents and subsidized insurance for people of modest means, and offered regular-priced insurance for everyone else. In addition to the individual mandate, it levied penalties on larger employers who did not provide health insurance to workers. It also established the Massachusetts Health Connector as an independent public agency to serve as an insurance marketplace, offering a wide array of private insurance plans to individuals and small businesses through its website.

The Massachusetts law was based on the notion of shared responsibility and it succeeded in almost every respect. Most notably, it brought the state's uninsured rate down to 2 percent in the first three years—that's near-universal coverage and closer to a fully insured population than any state had achieved in the nation's history. Many who wouldn't have had access to health insurance before the law were newly able to afford healthcare. One such patient was twenty-seven-year-old Jaclyn Michalos, who was diagnosed with breast cancer right after she got her insurance coverage. She worked in her family's restaurant and had no health insurance until the Health Connector came along. She explained, "If I didn't have health insurance, I would never have made an appointment with my doctor because of the cost. The cancer would have spread and I would not be alive today to tell you my story."[4]

The Massachusetts Health Connector received national attention, and the designers of the ACA wanted to build on its success. Let's look at how they did that.

THE ACA'S BALANCED DESIGN

The ACA's designers based the private insurance portion of the ACA on the Massachusetts model, intending to fix the rest of the country's individual market shortcomings with the same simple framework that Massachusetts had used: "shared responsibility" for individuals and employers, the healthcare industry (including insurers), and the government. This framework is embodied in the image of a three-legged stool, and the idea is simple: you need all three legs of the stool, or the system won't be balanced either politically or functionally.

Politically, Americans prefer solutions that incorporate individual responsibility with government assistance, so that programs are not just "handouts." Functionally, a balanced system ensures a broad risk pool for health insurance, meaning it covers the sick and the healthy, so that prices are kept under control. (Reminder: if only sick people buy insurance, prices become exorbitant.)

This balanced system incorporated several key elements: incentives to motivate people to sign up, consumer protections, fair pricing and cost containment initiatives, and a trustworthy place to shop for individual and small group coverage. Layered alongside all of this focus on the individual market was an expansion of the Medicaid program and other beneficial provisions that improved coverage for millions of Americans.

MOTIVATING PEOPLE TO SIGN UP

The ACA's individual market framework included a combination of incentives and penalties—a sort of "carrot and stick" approach—designed to encourage people to sign up for health insurance. Some of the incentives affected individuals and families, some affected companies. Subsidies to help pay for coverage were the biggest carrot used to inspire individuals to buy health insurance, while the biggest stick was the individual mandate, which would penalize those who still refused to buy insurance. This approach was needed to guarantee enough young and healthy people, "young invincibles," would buy health insurance, to keep the risk pool healthier and premiums lower.

The health insurance incentives were primarily tax subsidies designed to make insurance more affordable for lower- to moderate-income people who weren't able to get health insurance coverage through their jobs, but whose income was too high for Medicaid. This was significant for affordability: over 60 percent of people purchasing coverage in the individual market today benefit from these subsidies (including over 80 percent buying through exchanges).[5] The ACA also established other affordability measures, such as cost-sharing limits: it set an out-of-pocket maximum for most health insurance plans (including employer-sponsored), which meant that even for expensive medications or health emergencies, an individual in 2019 would never have to pay more than $7,900 per year (beyond their premium payments) and families would be capped at $15,800. Some insurance plans did not have an out-of-pocket limit before the ACA. By helping individuals minimize the cost of purchasing insurance, policymakers succeeded in motivating more people to sign up.

Meanwhile, predicting that some people still wouldn't buy into the new system, policymakers created the individual mandate, which was designed as a tax penalty for those who didn't buy health insurance even though they could afford it. The mandate reinforced the idea of shared responsibility and the importance of having a broad risk pool.

The mandate was also intended to eliminate the "free rider" problem. The phrase "free rider" is an economic term used to describe a group of people who get something without paying for it. In the case of healthcare, it's the people who don't have health insurance and show up in the emergency room for treatment. Hospitals have to provide them with a certain level of care, but are not compensated for it. However, even if uninsured people receive "free care" in the emergency room, the vast majority aren't trying to stick someone else with their medical bills. In fact, 76 percent of the uninsured believe that health insurance is something they need.[6] Most simply can't afford it. However, the fact remains that the health system has to absorb a large amount of uncompensated care, and the mandate was an effective way to make sure everyone pitched in.

PROTECTING CONSUMERS

Many of the ACA's key provisions were designed to protect consumers by setting national standards for health insurance coverage overall, though it focused primarily on the individual and small group health insurance markets. Before the ACA, there was tremendous state variation in the individual and small group markets, so a person living in Alabama, for instance, had dramatically different individual and small group market health insurance options than a person living in Massachusetts. After the ACA was passed, all health insurance sold to individuals and small businesses had to be high quality, meaning it had to include three main components (which I call "The Big Three"): 1) essential health benefits, 2) protections for people with pre-existing conditions, and 3) no annual or lifetime benefits caps. It also had to be priced fairly and be as affordable as possible.

1. Essential health benefits

The ACA mandated that all individual and small group market policies had to cover "essential health benefits," such as maternity care and mental healthcare. This was a big step forward for women's health. Prior to the ACA, 80 percent of individual policies excluded maternity coverage; all had to include the coverage once the ACA was implemented.

One of the ACA's goals was to address gaps like these, so it specified that health benefits must include at least ten categories of services—these were designated as "essential health benefits": ambulatory (outpatient) services, emergency room services, inpatient hospitalization, maternity care, mental health and substance abuse, prescriptions, rehabilitative and habilitative services and devices, laboratory services, preventive services (including chronic disease management), and pediatric dental and vision coverage.

Three of these benefits are more controversial than the others: maternity care, mental health/substance abuse care, and pediatric dental and vision coverage. They are prone to criticism because people who don't need these services and don't anticipate ever needing them believe they are subsidizing those who do. These three services were commonly left out of individual insurance plans before the ACA. If the ten essential health benefits requirement is ever repealed, I expect these services will be the first to be left out of plans, even though they don't make up a very big portion of the total cost of each plan—only about 5 percent. The three biggest pieces of healthcare spending, as shown below, are ambulatory (outpatient) services, hospitalization, and prescription drugs. (See figure 5.1.)

The coverage of birth control and maternity care remains especially controversial, and the debate over whether these services should be covered rages on. Apparently, many think it's unfair that they pay for services used only by women of childbearing age. And yet, these services benefit our society as a whole. Women may be only 50 percent of the current population, but we are responsible for delivering 100 percent of the future population. Maternity care helps ensure that we can safely give birth to healthy children. Similarly, though some women may choose not to use birth control for personal reasons, it is socially and fiscally responsible to make it accessible to everyone; the cost of birth control is far less than the cost of child support. (Maybe a rebranding from "birth control pills" to "child support expense control pills" would increase support for this coverage.)

FIGURE 5.1 Typical Relative Costs for the Essential Health Benefits Categories in the Commercial Market

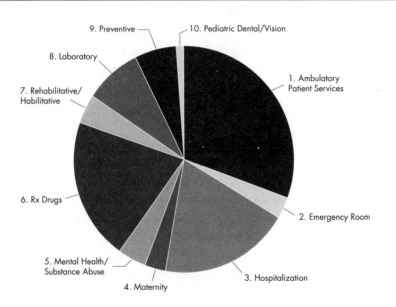

Source: Rebekah Bayram and Barbara Dewey, "Are Essential Health Benefits Here to Stay?," Milliman White Paper, March 2017, http://us.milliman.com/uploadedFiles/insight/2017/essential-health-benefits.pdf.

While the debate over which health benefits should be deemed "essential" continues, I think it's clear that many people buying health insurance don't know what they will need until they need it—even the need for maternity coverage can be an unexpected surprise, as it is for about half of pregnancies.[7] Take, for example, the story of former high school biology teacher Amy Tiller. After giving birth to twins, Amy was surprised to find out she didn't have maternity coverage for her third child, the reason being that she'd left her teaching job and bought insurance in the individual market, assuming it covered everything. When she discovered that it didn't, it was too late—there was a waiting period to be eligible to buy a rider to her policy for maternity coverage, which exceeded the length of her pregnancy. Before the ACA, her pregnancy was considered to be a preexisting condition, so coverage was either delayed (past the point of giving birth!) or denied.[8]

Amy was not alone—most people have a tough time understanding all of the fine print in insurance policies, which means they often don't know when benefits are excluded. Ensuring coverage for a comprehensive set of benefits addresses the unexpected and provides immeasurable peace of mind.

2. Protection for people with preexisting conditions

The ACA dramatically improved insurance practices regarding preexisting conditions. First, the ACA established an outright ban on excluding or charging more to people with preexisting conditions.[9] Second, through the use of a mechanism called risk adjustment, it curtailed the subtle economic tweaking that made plans unappealing to people with preexisting conditions.[10] Risk adjustment is a way to compensate insurers competing in the same risk pool for ending up with sicker patients. Under the ACA, insurers with healthier patients transfer funds to those with sicker patients. This compensation helped remove incentives for insurers to try to edge sicker patients out of their systems, so everyone's insurance plans improved.

A "preexisting condition" is a health condition that someone has before their health insurance goes into effect, and it includes a wide range of things, from serious conditions like cancer (even if it's cured) or heart disease, to more common conditions, like asthma, depression, and high blood pressure. Other examples include AIDS, arthritis, Crohn's disease, obesity, Parkinson's, stroke, domestic abuse, and gender dysphoria. Insurers know better than anyone how much it costs to treat a specific medical condition, so prior to the ACA insurers had policies that prevented more "expensive people" from enrolling with them. (There were six states, including Massachusetts, that guaranteed the sale of health insurance to all residents, but as noted earlier, that insurance tended to be very expensive.)

Thanks to the ACA, insurance companies now have to cover *everyone*, regardless of health status. And they can no longer charge sick people more.[11] Making this a law was monumental, benefiting just over half of nonelderly Americans (133 million people) who have preexisting conditions.[12] This includes adults and children who have a condition that would cause their premiums to be higher if the ACA weren't providing protection.[13] Twenty-seven percent of adult Americans have preexisting conditions that would leave them outright uninsurable if it weren't for the ACA.[14] These previously uninsurable conditions are more common among working-age women than men (partly due to pregnancy being considered "uninsurable" if a woman didn't already have insurance coverage). This means that protecting coverage for preexisting conditions is especially important for women's health.

Protecting people with preexisting conditions has turned out to be a very popular part of the ACA, once people realized its value during the ACA repeal attempts: over 75 percent of those surveyed in 2018 said that protecting people with preexisting conditions was "very important."[15] Repeated talk of repeal increased the salience of the issue, because people realized that something they had gained could be lost. The protections for people with preexisting conditions became a vote-defining issue during the midterm congressional elections in 2018. Since people with preexisting conditions make up so much of the US population, very few people wanted to go back to the bad old days of not having those protections.

3. No limits on coverage, annually or lifetime

Prior to the ACA, a person with a serious health condition like hemophilia could hit a *lifetime* limit of coverage and find themselves with no health insurance.[16] Over half of employer-sponsored insurance plans had lifetime limits that averaged roughly $5 million, but many were as low as $1 million or less.[17] Health plans with a lifetime limit would stop paying for an enrollee's healthcare expenses after they reached a set dollar amount of reimbursement over the entire life of the policy, potentially leaving the sickest patients responsible for extremely high costs. Enrollees could also hit an *annual* benefit limit where a health plan would stop paying for an enrollee's healthcare expenses after they reached a set dollar threshold each year—a typical amount was $500,000.[18]

The ACA prohibits *all* health plans from placing annual and lifetime dollar limits on the amount of health expenses they will cover. The good news is that this rule applies to employer-sponsored insurance, including mid- and large-size companies, as well as the individual marketplace. Annual and lifetime limits were among the most unpopular and contemptible practices in health insurance before they were banned by the ACA. The elimination of lifetime benefit caps helps upwards of twenty-five thousand people per year who would otherwise have maxed out their insurance benefit and had nowhere to turn.[19]

The elimination of lifetime limits did not raise premiums in a significant way.[20] Nevertheless, in 2017, the Republicans introduced the American Health Care Act, a bill to replace the ACA, which would have allowed these limits to be reintroduced.[21] It failed to pass. In fact, it was one of the most unpopular bills in decades, garnering only 29 percent support in national polls and no majority support in any state.[22] An enormous public outcry fought it back. Supporters of health coverage erupted in the streets in huge numbers, some with "die-ins," including coffins decorated with skulls and crossbones, theatrically demonstrating the link between the proposed bill and the deaths that would result from a mass loss of coverage as a consequence of the bill.

Now, since this aspect of the ACA remains intact, families can breathe more easily knowing that even if the worst-case health scenario happens, they know there's a dollar amount that they will never have to surpass in a given year, and they won't hit a lifetime limit on their benefits.

FAIR PRICING AND COST CONTAINMENT

Before the ACA, insurers in the individual and small group markets could differentiate their prices based on a person's gender, age, and health status. In fact, health insurers had penalized women for a long time by charging them higher premiums for individual market health insurance, presumably because they used more healthcare. As discussed above, they also charged people with preexisting conditions more than those without. These practices were eliminated by the ACA.

The ACA still allows insurers to charge older people more than younger people, but it limits the range of premiums to a three-to-one ratio, meaning they can charge people in the oldest age bracket only up to three times what they charge people in the youngest age bracket. Prior to the ACA, the ratio was not limited, and older Americans usually paid about five times as much in premiums.

The ACA also set rules to ensure that consumers were getting value for their healthcare dollar. The law requires insurers in the individual market to spend 80 percent of healthcare premiums on healthcare. (This is known as their medical loss ratio, or MLR.) The remaining 20 percent can be spent on administrative expenses and profit. Prior to the ACA, there were insurers in the individual market who spent only 60 percent of premiums on healthcare and took the rest as administration and profit. This took advantage of unsuspecting people who needed health insurance.

Lastly, to make high-quality healthcare more affordable, the ACA added new cost containment provisions. These provisions did not receive as much attention as the ACA's coverage elements and are beyond the scope of this book. They are important, nonetheless, because they are designed to move the healthcare system as a whole to a more affordable place. The ACA encouraged hospitals, physicians, and other healthcare providers to move away from fee-for-service payment by paying for value, not volume, through Accountable Care Organizations, bundled payments, and more. It targeted reducing preventable problems, like hospital-acquired infections or hospital readmissions, by penalizing hospitals with poor rates. Though great ideas, they have proven to be difficult to implement.

A TRUSTWORTHY PLACE TO SHOP

To bring all of this together and make buying insurance in the individual market easier, the ACA set up government-enabled health insurance exchanges modeled on the Massachusetts Health Connector. The exchanges provided people with a trustworthy place to buy individual coverage. Designed to foster a healthy competition on premiums among insurers, the exchanges allowed insurers to compete for individual consumer business on a level playing field.[23] By bringing some fairness and structure to the marketplace, the exchanges meant that health plan prices could be based more on the ideals of supply and demand, which would make health insurance more affordable.

Ultimately, the exchanges were intended to support consumers (anyone who needed to buy health insurance), and they had the potential to become the Travelocity of health insurance. People could go to an approved online exchange marketplace and make an "apples-to-apples" comparison across different insurance products at different tiers ("platinum," "gold," "silver," and "bronze") which varied by premium levels and amounts insurers would cover. In addition, exchange customers would be supported by call centers and online tools. Combined, these approaches could address the market failure issue of consumers having "imperfect information." Prior to the ACA, people who wanted to purchase a health plan needed to go through a broker, private marketplace, or insurance company. But that process was often confusing and inefficient—they experienced difficulty finding plans that matched their needs and budgets when searching sources one by one. The exchanges fixed this.

The exchanges were intended to be set up at the state level, but most states opted to be part of the federal exchange, Healthcare.gov. In 2019, only twelve states ran their own exchanges, but that included some large ones, such as California and New York. These state and federal exchanges are currently supporting over eleven million consumers nationwide and have served millions more since inception. Unfortunately, once Trump was elected, the federal government pulled back on its commitment to Healthcare.gov. Still, state exchanges remained invested in success. As a result, the twelve states running their own exchanges are better able to hold down prices and maintain higher enrollment than those that had been depending on the national exchange. This has led more states to pursue the launch of their own exchanges.

BEYOND THE INDIVIDUAL MARKET

In addition to reforming the individual insurance market, the ACA helped expand healthcare coverage in two other key areas. First, the ACA profoundly shifted the landscape by opening up Medicaid to millions more people. The biggest federal-level change to Medicaid since its inception, the ACA's Medicaid expansion accounts for about half of the ACA's coverage gains. The law required every state to extend Medicaid coverage to *all* of its citizen residents with incomes less than 138 percent of the federal poverty level (approximately $29,000 for a family of three)—including childless adults. This was a dramatic expansion of eligibility—before the ACA, only eighteen states covered parents whose incomes were at or above the federal poverty level.[24] However, a 2012 Supreme Court ruling ordered that the Medicaid expansion must be an option for states and not a requirement. As of mid-2019, fourteen states have not expanded. (More on this in chapter 6.)

Second, the ACA also allowed people with family coverage to keep their adult children on their insurance plan as "dependents" up until age twenty-six. This was an inexpensive and relatively easy way to expand coverage to over six million people, and it provides a whole lot of peace of mind to families.[25] It is one of the most popular provisions of the ACA.

THE ACA'S SHORTCOMINGS

The ACA has three major shortcomings. The first, and biggest, is that the ACA did not make its coverage affordable enough. This is one of the key reasons that over twenty-eight million people remain uninsured, and millions more defer needed healthcare treatments. The exchanges offered subsidies, but the subsidy amounts taper off at middle-income levels, which left many people having to pay the full cost of their insurance. Even people who have employer-sponsored health insurance coverage often struggle with high out-of-pocket costs and end up deferring needed healthcare (more on this in chapter 6). So, when something named the Affordable Care Act didn't solve the healthcare affordability problem, people were disappointed, to say the least.

The second is that it did not sufficiently address the rising costs of the healthcare system as a whole. It was focused on increasing access to healthcare, but ultimately our healthcare system needs to be affordable to be sustainable and ensure continued access.

The ACA's third shortcoming is that not enough people understood it. That is, not enough attention was dedicated to raising public awareness of the many benefits that accompanied the ACA. There are many people who are unaware of the financial assistance and significant provisions benefiting women. And most people certainly don't know about the shared responsibility (three-legged stool) framework. Without this context, it's easy to dislike the less popular ACA provisions (like the individual mandate) and to try to divorce them from the more popular provisions (like protection for preexisting conditions). But that makes the system go out of balance and undermines the ACA's coverage provisions.

The notion of balance is an important one. I've used the image of a three-legged stool throughout this chapter. As it relates to the individual mandate, another image comes to mind, and it's one that every parent struggles to enforce with their children: that of a well-balanced meal. As tempting as it may be, you can't just eat dessert (offer health insurance to all) to stay healthy—you have to eat your broccoli too (accept the individual mandate, or some other form of requirement to pay into the healthcare system).

UPSETTING THE BALANCE

The ACA was designed to achieve a delicate balance of coverage and affordability in the individual market through its three-legged stool model. Unfortunately, the ACA's elusive balance has been upset by a series of politically motivated efforts to repeal the law. The ACA has faced attacks ever since it was signed into law. There were immediate attempts to repeal it. In fact, there were more than fifty such attempts while President Obama was in office. They didn't prevail, however. There were also numerous court challenges which began during his term and continue to the present day.

The ACA repeal attempts became a rallying cry for many Republicans running for election in 2016. And yet, just after Trump took office, it became clear that Americans didn't want the ACA repealed without a suitable replacement. The consumer protections were firmly in place and the coverage gains had taken hold. Most Americans didn't want to go backward. The problem was that the "replacement" options were either not fleshed out or were too draconian—they would drastically weaken one or more legs of the stool and upset the ACA's balance.

These repeated repeal efforts detract from opportunities to introduce legislation to improve the ACA. No law is perfect from the outset, and the ACA would have benefited from adjustments. A similar process took place in Massachusetts; legislators had to refine the health reform law after it was passed, and they were able to make the necessary changes thanks to a cooperative political environment. Attempts to repeal the ACA have also created tremendous uncertainty in the marketplace, both for consumers and insurers. One state exchange director told me how he had to start every talk he gave to potential customers during 2017 with the reassuring statement, "We're still here!"

Short of repealing the ACA, the Trump administration has taken repeated actions to undermine the law. The most significant of these was done in conjunction with the Republican-controlled House and Senate: the repeal of the individual mandate penalty in late 2017. The Congressional Budget Office estimates that it will result in premium increases of 10 percent in the individual market and will cause up to thirteen million people to drop out of the market.

The Trump administration also took steps to undermine the advertising, outreach, and enrollment activities of Healthcare.gov, which reduced the number of people signing up for individual insurance. Since exchanges experience a high degree of turnover in their customer base as people's jobs and benefit status change, they continually need to attract new enrollees to keep risk pools large and premiums affordable. Additionally, consumers won't know they may be eligible for subsidies if no one tells them. Helping individuals and families enroll in the right insurance program for them requires ongoing advertising and outreach, so cutting federal funding in those areas results in fewer enrollments across the board—meaning more people are uncovered, undercovered, or paying excessively high rates for their coverage. One study showed that 2.5 million people could have received a subsidy if they'd purchased through the exchange.[26] State exchanges have remained invested in outreach efforts, but the federal exchange, Healthcare.gov, has significantly reduced funding for these activities, leaving many folks unaware of—and therefore unable to access—the benefits of the ACA.

Finally, the Trump administration released new rules in 2018 to allow people to purchase health coverage that is not compliant with the ACA. This undermines the ACA and its exchange marketplaces by potentially siphoning off healthy people into alternative health insurance options. The worst of these options are the skimpy, "short-term limited duration" plans that were originally meant to fill coverage gaps. These plans are subject to virtually none of the ACA's protections. The Trump administration allowed these plans to extend to twelve months and made them renewable, essentially offering a replacement for ACA-compliant individual market plans. Experts are concerned that those who purchase these types of plans will be in for an unpleasant surprise when they get sick and realize their plan's shortcomings. In addition, short-term plans are low value: as much as half of what insurers collect in premiums goes to their administration and profit, not enrollees' health.[27] Contrast this with ACA-compliant plans, where at least 80 percent of premiums go to health. So, although short-term plans are somewhat cheaper, they offer far fewer benefits: fewer than a third of short-term plans reviewed recently cover prescription drugs and not one single plan covers maternity care.[28] They also have annual benefit limits, which are illegal for ACA-compliant plans.[29]

Since, by law, short-term plans cannot be sold on public exchanges, they are mostly marketed online or through mailers, often in dishonest or misleading ways. Buried in the fine print may be dollar coverage limits, including for specific line items. One unfortunate man in Washington, DC, who believed he was covered for up to $750,000 of care including surgery, found that because of these line-item coverage limits ($2,500 for surgeon fees; $1,000 per day for an inpatient stay) his short-term insurance only had to pay $11,780 of his $212,000 bill.[30]

Moreover, the availability of these plans, in combination with the repeal of the individual mandate penalty, may lead to an exodus of healthy people from the individual insurance markets, destabilizing these marketplaces and leading to a spike in their premiums.

Efforts to undermine the ACA are subtle and insidious. As noted earlier, millions are expected to lose coverage due to the repeal of the individual mandate penalty. But the other factors, though perhaps less directly harmful, do create additional problems. While eliminating advertising funding or offering short-term plans may seem like small enough moves by themselves, they have large and sometimes unpredictable repercussions, and they all add up.

Beyond politics, there are the challenges of the larger market forces affecting the individual health insurance marketplace, including the rising cost of healthcare. The individual marketplace has always been less protected from these forces, and it also has more ups and downs than the group insurance market, due in part to the frequently changing circumstances of its customer base. These fundamental facts make the individual market very expensive for people who aren't subsidized.[31] Insurers have tried to keep premiums down to stay competitive in the marketplace. One of the ways they have done this is by shifting the costs from premiums to cost-sharing, especially deductibles.[32]

Why are individual marketplace premiums so high and rising? First, individual market enrollees lack the power of employers who negotiate on behalf of their employees. But a whole host of other factors have contributed to increasing costs for consumers, including the rising cost of medical care overall, which in turn includes the increasing costs of hospital stays, physician visits, and prescription drugs. When the insurer has to pay more for these things, it has to increase premiums.

Also, rising premiums cause rising premiums. This isn't a typo. It's a vicious self-fulfilling cycle: every time premiums rise, a few more healthy people decide that even though insurance protects them, the price is higher than they are willing to pay. When these healthy people don't purchase insurance, the subscriber pools become sicker, insurance companies have to pay out more in claims per person, and then they have to raise premiums to cover these costs. Rinse and repeat.

Rising premiums on the individual market have come under great scrutiny, although these increases are actually *lower* than they likely would have been in the absence of the ACA.[33] Nonetheless, a March 2018 poll by the Kaiser Family Foundation found that 75 percent to 80 percent of individual market enrollees were worried about their co-pays, deductibles, and premiums rising to be so high that they wouldn't be able to afford the healthcare they need.[34]

This raises tremendous concerns—people need this insurance. The individual market cannot solve this problem on its own—it needs help.

I TOOK THE JOB at the Massachusetts Health Connector because I wanted to work on a cause that I passionately believed in—expanding health insurance coverage to those like Jaclyn Michalos who didn't have any. I also wanted *everyone* to have access to health insurance, regardless of their health status. I still believe in these causes, and working on the ACA has allowed me to work on these issues at a national level.

The ACA made a good start to improving the individual market and expanding coverage, but it hasn't accomplished enough. It was launched with great fanfare, and relative to its potential and those high expectations, it underperformed. This left it vulnerable to attacks, including efforts to repeal the law. It pains me to see it, given how Massachusetts was able to get to near-universal coverage with the same framework. The fact that the ACA fell short is helping to spur the enthusiasm for the universal coverage movement today.

The ACA's shortcomings are not insurmountable. They could be addressed with some fairly simple fixes, and a commitment to funding them (more on this in chapters 10 and 11). And, in spite of its shortcomings, the ACA was a huge improvement over the prior world of the individual insurance market where there were some terrible insurance practices.

At this time of political peril for the ACA, I see two things. The first is that we cannot go backward—we must move forward. This means that we cannot allow the ACA to be repealed, or further undermined. The second is that to move forward, we need to fix the ACA. Later I will argue that we need to go even further than that to truly establish healthcare as a right. But repairing and enhancing the current ACA is a significant next step that we should take.

Even though the ACA didn't go far enough, we can't lose sight of its accomplishments and the shared responsibility framework upon which it was built. We have made tremendous gains through the ACA. I started writing this book because I wanted to show people how truly important the steps we've taken are, to raise awareness and help us all understand what makes progress possible. The gains we've made deserve to be protected. Better yet, they should be expanded upon, because too many people have been left uncovered.

■ ■ ■ ■ ■ ■

CHAPTER 6

LEFT UNCOVERED

Of all the forms of inequality, injustice in health
care is the most shocking and inhumane.

—DR. MARTIN LUTHER KING JR.[1]

SOME TWENTY-EIGHT MILLION AMERICANS—9 percent of our population—currently have no health insurance. That number includes more
than four million children, which is a moral outrage that does not receive
nearly enough national attention. For a country where most believe healthcare to be a right, the percentage of uninsured is shockingly high, and worse
yet, the number is starting to rise.[2]

Growing up in a middle-class family where my father had a job with
health insurance, I never experienced being uninsured. In fact, I took the
coverage our family had for granted. But when I got my first job at the
YWCA, a nonprofit with an all-female staff, I worked with single mothers
who worried about their young adult children who didn't have coverage. I
began to notice the fear, uncertainty, and stress that comes from being uninsured. I also heard from family members who were concerned about my
cousins who were facing troubling health issues, including substance abuse,
without insurance. I could see these issues taking a toll.

How did we end up with a system that fails so many? Mostly because our
patchwork quilt of health insurance coverage grew piece by piece, and not
comprehensively. It resulted from a series of reactions to historical circumstances, including market failures and limited political opportunities. Hop-
ing for a win, and knowing that political leaders feared backlash from the
insurance industry and others, activists would push for one piece, as AIDS
activists did with the Ryan White CARE Act of 1990, which provided coverage for needy people with HIV/AIDS, rather than universal healthcare.

Who are the uninsured? They are the thirty-somethings working in the gig economy, driving for Uber or making Amazon's deliveries. They are the twenty-somethings waiting tables, whose parents don't have an employer-sponsored insurance plan to add them to. They are the women who clean houses, work as personal care attendants, or are preschool teachers. The majority of uninsured people are low income, but contrary to stereotypes, the majority of uninsured people *are working*. And for those people lucky enough to be working and have employer-sponsored insurance, they are just one job loss away from having no coverage. This is an uneasy feeling for many.

The uninsured tend to be millennials—most are between the ages of twenty-six and thirty-five and earn a household income lower than $36,000 per year.[3] Most have jobs or live in a family with at least one employed person.[4] People of color are at a higher risk of being uninsured, as are undocumented immigrants (who are often ineligible for Medicaid or purchasing a marketplace plan).[5] Over a quarter of the uninsured in the US are actually eligible for Medicaid or the Children's Health Insurance Program but are not signed up.[6]

When health insurance is unaffordable, people become uninsured. In fact, the biggest reason that people are uninsured is due to cost. The cost is high and growing, dramatically outpacing the growth in wages. This affects people across the income spectrum. In fact, the premiums for family coverage now cost more than a typical mortgage payment, and the premiums for individual coverage cost more than a car payment. Life changes like divorce, graduation, and death of family members, as well as giving birth, switching jobs, and experiencing income fluctuations, all contribute to uninsurance. A brief lapse in coverage is risky, but two-thirds of people who are currently uninsured have lacked coverage for more than a year; they are in an especially precarious situation.[7] Not only are the long-term uninsured living with no protection against catastrophic medical bills, they also aren't likely to be taking steps to detect and prevent more serious illnesses.

Even though most people think about being uninsured as a financial issue, if you look at it from another perspective, being uninsured is a chronic condition. Like diabetes or lupus, uninsurance amplifies the negative effects of other diseases, worsens quality of life, and ultimately increases likelihood of death. People without health insurance are more than six times as likely as those with health insurance to go without needed care due to cost. They are also more than four times as likely to have no usual source of care, which limits doctors' ability to recommend preventive measures and other care based on knowledge of their patients' health history.[8]

These numbers directly translate into mortality.

During the height of the GOP's efforts to repeal the ACA in 2017, one Republican lawmaker famously said: "Nobody dies because they don't have access to health care."[9] Nothing could be further from the truth. People without insurance are at a 3–41 percent increased risk of death. And an estimated 26,000 adults between the ages of twenty-five and sixty-five died because they didn't have health insurance in 2010.[10] In its groundbreaking report on the uninsured, the Institute of Medicine concluded that working-age Americans without health insurance are more likely to "receive too little medical care and receive it too late, be sicker and die sooner, and receive poorer care when they are in the hospital even for acute situations like a motor vehicle crash."[11]

Because uninsured people receive less preventive care and fewer screenings, their downstream costs and health consequences can balloon as conditions go undetected for longer. Women without health insurance have a 30–50 percent higher risk of dying from breast cancer because it is detected later, and when it is detected they receive less extensive treatment.[12]

Likewise, common chronic diseases such as cardiovascular disease, kidney disease, HIV, and mental illness diseases can be exacerbated by a lack of insurance.[13] Diabetics, for example, need to monitor their health with periodic lab tests and physical exams. But a quarter of uninsured diabetics go without checkups for multiple years.[14]

Uninsured patients also receive inadequate acute care (hospital) services. They are less inclined to seek it (knowing that they will be sent a bill that they are often unable to pay), and the quality of care they receive is below average. This is because hospital staff know the care they provide to the uninsured is likely to be uncompensated. So, they offer fewer needed services, and are less likely to admit an uninsured person to inpatient care. This translates into a higher-than-average risk of death during hospitalization or immediately following discharge.[15] The resulting outcome disparities are staggering—one study found that uninsured car crash victims are 37 percent more likely to die than their insured counterparts.[16]

The death of Amy Vilela's daughter, Shalynne, is a tragic example of this outrageous situation. Shalynne was enrolling in nursing school and was in between insurance coverage when she went to the emergency room with a pain in her leg. Because she appeared to be uninsured, the hospital sent her home. "They're telling her it's going to be very expensive, she can leave now, there's the door, it won't cost her anything," Vilela said. "They want us to see if we can get her on our insurance."[17] The pain worsened, and a few weeks later she returned to the hospital and died of a blood clot that had traveled from her leg to her groin. Outraged at a healthcare system that allows people like her daughter to die because she fell between the coverage cracks, Vilela decided to run for Congress in Nevada as a health-care-for-all activist.[18]

WHY ARE THERE SO MANY UNINSURED?

Despite the wide variety of coverage programs in the US, there is no universal solution. The high percentage of uninsured people has been a priority for some lawmakers for decades, but their patchwork approach to a fix hasn't been enough. This leaves bare spots in the coverage quilt, and they are starting to grow. There are two main components of this growth: the erosion of existing patches and the gaps between the patches that were never closed and are now widening.

To recap, the American healthcare coverage quilt consists of four main patches: Medicare, which covers the elderly; employer-sponsored insurance, which covers most of the working-age population and their children; Medicaid for those with no employer-sponsored insurance and very low incomes; and the individual marketplace, or "nongroup" insurance, which is available for purchase by those with no employer-sponsored insurance and moderate to higher incomes. However, these patches do not always work as intended. If they did, the system should be equipped to cover everyone who wants insurance, regardless of income. The designers of the ACA certainly tried to cover the bare patches and get more Americans insured. Unfortunately, things didn't turn out quite as they planned.

The biggest wrench thrown into the gears of the ACA's coverage expansion plan happened with a landmark Supreme Court decision in 2012.[19] As mentioned, the ACA initially required states to provide Medicaid to *every* citizen with incomes under 138 percent of the federal poverty level (about $29,000 for a family of three)[20]—for most states, this was an expansion of their Medicaid program. States that didn't would forfeit their federal Medicaid funding. But the Supreme Court decided that this was "coercive" and struck it from the law.

After the decision, some states expanded their Medicaid program, and some exercised their newfound right not to. The states that expanded Medicaid enjoyed significant gains in coverage, especially for childless adults who were often excluded from the program before the ACA. These states also received generous federal funding for the expansion population, covering nearly their entire cost. As of early 2019, thirty-six states (plus Washington, DC) have expanded Medicaid.[21]

The governors and legislators of the fourteen states that have not yet expanded Medicaid have harmed their citizens, particularly those with low incomes. Eleven of these states provide no coverage for childless adults and provide Medicaid only to parents who earn less than $10,000 a year.[22] Texas and Alabama win the race to the bottom. If you live in either of those states, you must earn less than $3,800 per year and be a parent in a family of three to qualify for Medicaid; childless adults are ineligible.[23]

It gets worse. Some people were left completely in the cold, without even being able to get exchange subsidies. This is because the drafters of the ACA, not anticipating that the Medicaid expansion would be altered by the US Supreme Court, set the threshold for the individual market subsidies at 100 percent of the federal poverty level (FPL), assuming that anybody with income less than that would receive Medicaid. But some of those people don't receive Medicaid because the states they live in chose not to expand the program, even with federal money to help. The people most harmed by a state not expanding Medicaid are the poorest of the uninsured, those with incomes below the federal poverty level. They have fallen into a coverage gap.[24]

An essay in *Unequal Coverage* tells the story of Ana, a thirty-six-year-old Texan who is the daughter of Mexican immigrants.[25] Ana falls in Texas' Medicaid coverage gap. She is working a series of part-time retail jobs while also caring for her mother who has dementia. She is in an impossible situation: none of her jobs offer health insurance, she doesn't earn enough to qualify for an exchange subsidy, and she earns too much to qualify for the Texas Medicaid program, which is cruelly insufficient in any case. At one point while caring for her mother she actually qualified for indigent care, but the process of applying for this type of coverage was degrading. "I don't pay a dime, but I do pay a price," she said, when describing the police-like scrutiny she received when seeking this coverage. "They want you to stay down because if you advance, you're not worthy of that coverage."

Like Ana, many working Americans are also feeling the squeeze of unaffordable health insurance. Premiums for family coverage exceed the average cost of a mortgage ($997 per month vs. $758 per month in 2017).[26] As I discussed in chapter 4, the number of firms offering employer-sponsored insurance is declining, as is the percentage of costs that these plans cover. That throws more employees and their families into the individual insurance market, often without subsidies, or leaves them underinsured.[27]

Reporter Sarah Kliff tells the story of one such family that has "chosen" to be uninsured due to the sky-high prices of family coverage, even for a plan with a $5,000 deductible.[28] The story haunts Sarah because the parents recently had to make a tough choice when the poison control center told them to take their two-year-old daughter to the emergency room due to the Dramamine pills she had swallowed. The girl's mother, Lindsay Clark, already had an unpaid bill of $1,200 from her last trip to the emergency room. Lindsay said, "I'm weighing my options. She could have a seizure at any moment. It felt terrible, as a parent, to be in the position of having to do that." Lindsay and her husband decided to park outside the emergency room, administer the recommended antidote themselves (activated charcoal), and wait to see if their daughter would have seizures. They got lucky this time—the antidote worked and they took Lindsay home.

GROWING NUMBER OF UNDERINSURED

There's another healthcare problem simmering in the US: more people are becoming "underinsured," which means they are spending 5–10 percent of their income toward out-of-pocket healthcare expenses. There isn't really a recommended amount to spend on healthcare. However, median out-of-pocket healthcare spending in nonelderly US households is $800 per year, and median household income is about $59,000 annually, so out-of-pocket healthcare spending is often about 1.5 percent of income. This isn't a super-precise number, but it can be useful for comparison.

Underinsured people have health insurance, but their plans are nearly useless: either the cost-sharing is sky high or the coverage is extremely limited, or both.[29] Similar to being uninsured, many of them delay seeking care due to cost. Forty-one million Americans—28 percent of working-age adults—now qualify as underinsured. This is a big increase from 12 percent of working-age adults in 2003. It includes a whopping 25 percent of people with health insurance through their jobs, and 42 percent of people with individual market coverage.

The biggest culprit in this rise in underinsurance is the fact that cost-sharing (especially through deductibles) has been increasing rapidly over recent years. As described in chapter 4, rising deductibles pose one of the greatest threats to insurance affordability. In fact, deductibles are growing eight times faster than wages are.[30] (In 2003, 1 percent of private plans had a deductible of $3,000 or higher. By 2016, 13 percent did.)[31] Even smaller deductibles can be a problem—at least half of the workforce has a deductible of $1,000 or more. And yet, half of households have less than $1,000 in savings.[32] Almost half of underinsured adults who had trouble paying their medical bills said that they have used up all of their savings to pay those bills.

High deductibles can impact health. Just like the uninsured, people who are underinsured will often go without needed care because it's too expensive, and their care-seeking behavior bears this out: uninsured patients are 38 percent more likely than the well-insured to delay seeking emergency care for a heart attack, while the underinsured are 21 percent more likely to delay seeking care.[33] The underinsured are essentially in the same situation or worse than that of the uninsured until they reach their deductible (except for services exempt from the deductible, such as screenings and primary care visits.) If you are *uninsured* and need a $1,000 procedure, you owe $1,000. If you are *insured* by a plan with a high deductible and need a $1,000 procedure, you still owe $1,000, only in this case you have less money in the bank because you've been paying premiums.

The largest recent growth in the underinsured has been among those with employer-sponsored insurance: they now account for over half of the underinsured population, with the biggest growth coming from larger companies. However, people who purchase health insurance in the individual market are still the most likely to be underinsured.[34]

The reemergence of skimpy insurance plans is also contributing to rising underinsurance. Although this isn't part of the formal definition, I like to include skimpy plans under the category of underinsurance. Plans sold on exchanges and through employers should cover most needed services, as required by law. However, as discussed in chapter 5, short-term insurance plans have been creeping their way back into the market, with their penetration accelerating after the Trump administration loosened regulations on them. Some states have stepped in to regulate these plans in a few ways, including outlawing them or limiting their duration, but most haven't done anything yet.

Although the ACA increased the coverage offered by health plans and ensured that coverage is available to anyone, this came at a price. Higher cost-sharing and, consequently, higher underinsurance, are part of the price

Americans currently pay in order to get comprehensive benefits and have access to coverage when we have a preexisting condition. Unfortunately, this hurts some of our most vulnerable people. Of those who are ill and have high healthcare expenses, more than one-third are underinsured. This is compounded by the fact that 61 percent of the underinsured have low incomes.[35]

While a comprehensive healthcare coverage and affordability solution is what we ultimately need, we should put pressure now on states to anticipate the proliferation of skimpy plans and take action to protect consumers from these and other forms of underinsurance.

THE IMPACT ON WOMEN AND CHILDREN

The ACA's results have included some good news for working-age women: their rates of uninsurance have improved since the law was passed, dropping from 19 percent in 2013 to 11 percent in 2017.[36] Women are actually more likely to be insured than men. However, some women are more likely to be left without coverage.

Those who earn less than the federal poverty level or have no high school diploma, single mothers, Latinas, and noncitizens have higher rates of uninsurance, in some cases double that of the US average.[37] There are many low-income women who fall in the Medicaid coverage gap described above: they often don't have employer-sponsored insurance but they earn too much to qualify for Medicaid and not enough to afford individual market coverage. Women living in states that did not expand Medicaid experience higher rates of uninsurance too.[38] Texas has the dubious distinction of being the worst state in this regard: nearly one out of every five working-age women in Texas does not have health insurance.

Being underinsured disproportionately affects women. This is not because of the rate of underinsurance, which is about the same for men and women. It's because women are more likely to delay or forgo needed care because of affordability issues, and are more likely to be burdened by medical bills due in large part to the fact that they earn less money than men do.[39] These affordability issues are exacerbated by the fact that women tend to use the healthcare system more frequently and therefore have higher out-of-pocket costs than men. Skimpy insurance plans often exclude coverage for services that women use, but even ACA-compliant plans can leave out important services for women, such as maternity coverage for dependents, abortion coverage, and some forms of contraceptives.[40]

Another area that affects women greatly, given their ongoing role as care-givers of children, is the rate of uninsurance for children. More than four million children in the US, or about 5 percent of children, are uninsured.[41] This is a sizable decrease from 1997, when 14 percent of children were un-insured. However, it is still unconscionable that children must suffer because our nation can't figure out how to cover them.

Uninsured children have worse health outcomes, period. That should be justification enough to ensure universal coverage for them. But there are financial upsides as well: studies show that children who were covered by Medicaid had an increase in college attendance and earnings potential. Moreover, the government recoups 56 cents out of every dollar it spends to cover children through increased tax revenues, because beneficiaries are later more likely to receive higher income and less likely to be eligible for the earned income tax credit.[42] And insurance for teenagers can reduce un-planned pregnancies because the health system provides health education and contraceptives. Without these services, the cycle of un- and underinsur-ance is more likely to start all over again.

Plus, most kids don't use that much healthcare, and insuring the aver-age child costs about half as much as insuring the average adult.[43] Despite this, states vary tremendously in who they cover in their CHIP program. Every state has its own income standards for people to be able to enroll in the Medicaid and CHIP programs, but states tend to be more generous to children than adults. If family income is too high to be eligible for a state's Medicaid program, the CHIP program often covers children up to a higher eligibility level, which again varies by state.[44] The upper income limit ranges from $36,365 for a family of three in North Dakota, to just over $84,000 for a family of three in New York.[45]

Another major determinant of who's covered relates to who signs up for the program. Researchers estimate that 62–72 percent of uninsured children are actually eligible for Medicaid or CHIP,[46] but don't get enrolled because of confusion, misinformation, and other barriers. For example, 21 percent of low-income parents incorrectly believe their income is too high for their children to be eligible for Medicaid or CHIP, and 51 percent of parents whose children aren't currently enrolled think that enrolling would be "somewhat" or "very" hard.[47] In addition, one-third of Spanish-speaking parents believe they cannot afford Medicaid or CHIP, and yet both pro-grams are virtually free.[48]

Let's not place blame on the parents or caregivers, though. Many have stressful, immediate life concerns and other significant challenges that preclude them from becoming well versed in complex subjects like Medicaid and CHIP eligibility. And conveying that information can be *incredibly* difficult. Many potential Medicaid members don't know what Medicaid is, or that they could be covered by it. Despite the efforts that many states have made, some people don't receive or understand the message.

The Children's Health Insurance Program Reauthorization Act of 2009 (CHIPRA) attempted to increase enrollment of eligible children into Medicaid and CHIP by creating innovative strategies like "express lane" eligibility, which enables states to flag information from state income taxes and public programs such as school lunch programs and Head Start.[49] This information is then automatically sent to Medicaid or CHIP to help determine which children might need to be enrolled or renewed.[50] Unfortunately, express lane eligibility hasn't gained much traction;[51] currently only eight states have active programs.[52] That's because the program is built around the current system that requires eligibility verification, interagency communication, and public knowledge. In sum, there are too many administrative barriers.

Given all these barriers, the best way to care for children is with a government-sponsored universal coverage system for those under eighteen. A significant gain in coverage could be attained by automatically enrolling children in public health insurance when they are born, then requiring parents to opt out of it if they want them to be covered by private insurance. Instead, there is an expectation that parents will enroll their children in their employer-sponsored insurance, or into Medicaid or CHIP if employer-sponsored insurance is unavailable or too expensive. Putting that burden on parents means that a lot of children slip through the cracks.

In sum, the benefits to this country of insuring children—including teenagers—extend far beyond tax revenues, to improved economic participation, housing security, health, happiness, and future insurance coverage. Our country is full of promising children who won't end up in a position that reflects their abilities because their family can't afford to meet their basic needs, including healthcare.

UNCOMPENSATED CARE

In 1986, Congress passed a law called the Emergency Medical Treatment and Active Labor Act that required emergency rooms to evaluate and treat anyone who sought care from them, making them a major provider of uncompensated care. This requirement gave people who fell ill in the streets somewhere to turn. The total value of this care is substantial, despite the fact that uninsured people typically receive fewer and lower quality healthcare services in hospitals. Because three-fourths of care provided to the uninsured is not paid for (uncompensated), it places a major strain on our healthcare delivery system's finances. These costs fall mostly on the healthcare providers in low-income communities who can least afford to pay them.

Unfortunately, this law inadvertently created the "free rider problem" I described in the previous chapter: people can "choose" to not purchase insurance and show up for free care in the emergency room when they need it. But someone must pay for these expensive healthcare services. If we don't make healthcare a right in the US, we have three options: (1) we undo the law and leave uninsured people on the street to fend for themselves, (2) we require our healthcare deliverers to provide uncompensated care, or (3) we require people to pay for health insurance. The ACA's drafters thought the third option was the best idea and built the individual mandate into the law. As a result, uncompensated care costs decreased: In 2013, before the individual mandate went into effect, uncompensated care cost the system $85 billion.[53] In the first five years after the law went into effect, uncompensated care costs in hospitals fell by $12 billion, a 30 percent decrease.[54]

In spite of this, the individual mandate was the law's least popular (and potentially most misunderstood) provision, and its penalty has since been repealed. Many believe that the US government does not have the right to require people to purchase something, even though we do this in other areas. For instance, we require all drivers to have auto insurance. That said, nobody likes being forced to purchase anything, especially when it's as expensive as a health insurance plan. Some who opposed the individual mandate claimed they "never" use healthcare services. Others said that if they do need healthcare, they would be willing to pay out of pocket.

Here's the problem: Even if you have never used healthcare services, you will need to in the future. Anyone can find themselves a consumer of healthcare on any given, unlucky day, and the system will be ready for them, insured or not. I found myself in precisely this situation while I was writing this book; I slipped on a wet jet bridge while boarding an airplane, broke my ankle badly, was rushed to the emergency room and had to have surgery—an unexpected expense of $50,000. I was extremely lucky to be insured. Most of us can't afford to pay these types of medical bills out of pocket, which is why three-quarters of these bills go unpaid for uninsured people.

Unless you have a lot of money saved, being uninsured puts the health system at risk of having to absorb your uncompensated care. Even though most people pay more in premiums than they receive in care, which is justifiably frustrating, what is even more frustrating is when others must reimburse the care that someone else receives. Since emergency departments are not legally allowed to turn people away, hospitals must find a way to offset these increased costs, typically by charging more for those who are insured. If someone says it's unfair that they are required to purchase health insurance, ask them to consider who should pay their medical bills if they slip tomorrow and need a $50,000 operation to repair their broken ankle.

Finally, to come full circle, it's worth remembering that the burden of uncompensated care is borne not only by the health system, but by the uninsured people themselves. One study shows that a hospital admission is associated with an increase in unpaid bills of over $6,000 for the uninsured, compared to about $300 for the insured. These bills translate into adverse financial outcomes like reduced credit scores and bankruptcy,[55] and they also cause tremendous stress.

OUR CURRENT PATCHWORK system of health coverage straddles the line between public and private insurance, and it has left millions uninsured and millions more underinsured. The fact that most insurance is bought and sold by private individuals and companies presents a conundrum: we are so invested in having the private market provide healthcare that it is hard to see another way of doing things. Many believe that the private market's impact on society as a whole is justification for a higher degree of government involvement, to rein in the market's excesses and to address market failures. Yet many others believe government involvement decreases the freedom and efficiency of the private market. Unfortunately, this unresolved conflict in healthcare is causing needless anxiety, suffering, and deaths, all of which would be alleviated if healthcare were a right in the US.

Furthermore, what does it say about our country when barriers like uninsurance stack the deck against children as soon as they are born, regardless of their capabilities? Americans champion the free market because it is supposed to allow the hardest-working, highest achievers to succeed. If America wants to live up to its ideal of being a meritocracy, then we need to address these issues, including insuring all of our children.

As I'll explain in the final part of this book, there are ways to cover more people by finding a balance, without having to completely overhaul the system. People should have access to proper medical care, and the fact that 12 percent of Americans under age sixty-five lack health insurance is an injustice. We can, and must, do better.

CHAPTER 7

COVERAGE ALONE ISN'T ENOUGH

Unaddressed social and emotional stressors are often
at the root of patients' health struggles.

—ELIZABETH BRADLEY and LAUREN TAYLOR,
public health experts[1]

M Y HUSBAND AND I have been raising our three children in one of the most diverse cities in the country. Somerville, Massachusetts, is a microcosm of the US, racially and economically, thanks to many factors, including its wide variety of housing and its proximity to Boston. It has long been home to groups of immigrants from dozens of countries as well as longtime residents who have reached the middle class. Take a walk down Broadway, a main street near where I live, and you will see an Indian grocery store, a Haitian restaurant, a karate studio, pizza shops, and a new brew pub. Sprinkled throughout the mixed-income neighborhoods of triple-deckers and single family homes are writers, artists, restaurant workers, house cleaners, firefighters, small business owners, and entrepreneurs. As a parent and volunteer in the public schools, I've seen firsthand how people's health and well-being are affected by multiple factors, including stress levels, housing conditions, and economic opportunities. And from the people I know who must work too many jobs to make ends meet, to those who enjoy a comfortable level of professional success, we all share a common goal of having a safe, healthy community in which to live.

Numerous studies show that our health and well-being aren't impacted only by our access to medical care; they are also affected by a wide range of factors, such as socioeconomic status (including education level and employment), our social support networks, race, and our physical environment.

These nonmedical factors are called the "social determinants of health" and they are foundational to our well-being. If the US health insurance system is like a "quilt of coverage," then the social determinants are the underlying bedframe. Complex and interlocking, they need to be included in discussions about healthcare as a right. If the ultimate goal is to improve our health and well-being, it is critical to think beyond just access to healthcare and shift our mind-set to creating a culture of health.

Health is defined as "a state of complete physical, mental, and social well-being."[2] Foundational to our health are certain internal, *individual* determinants, such as our biology and our behavior. For example, we are born with certain genetic risk factors that we cannot control, such as a propensity for heart disease. But we can control behaviors that might mitigate this risk factor, such as diet and exercise.

Just as important to our health are the external, *social* determinants of health, such as education and housing. The availability and quality of these determinants are driven by societal factors that are mostly beyond our individual control but can be influenced through collective action. (See figure 7.1.)

FIGURE 7.1 Health Is Determined by Multiple Internal and External Factors beyond Healthcare

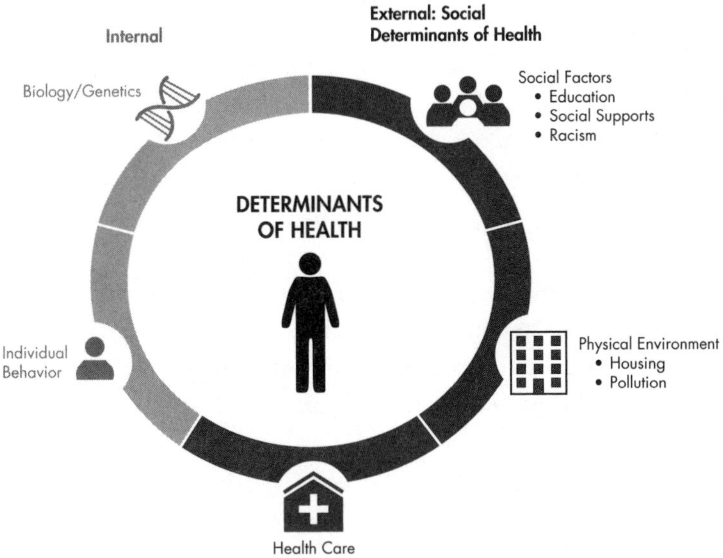

Source: Day Health Strategies, as informed by Edwin Choi, Juhan Sonin, "Determinants of Health," goinvo, https://www.goinvo.com/vision/determinants-of-health.

Looking at health in this holistic way, it becomes clear that access to healthcare is a necessary, but not sufficient, component of our individual health. Access to healthcare is important—it can make a difference between life and premature death. But so can other nonmedical factors. The nonmedical components of health include individual-level "social needs" (like friendship), and societal-level "social determinants" (like inadequate education or housing, or too much pollution) that must be addressed upstream at the public policy level, through some combination of education, social services, public health, workforce, and infrastructure initiatives.

The same holds true for the health of the entire population; access to healthcare is necessary, but not sufficient. Population health is very much driven by the social determinants of health. The inequities that permeate the social determinants (such as unequal educational opportunities or impoverished communities) are perpetuated in the healthcare system, both in terms of access to healthcare and in the quality of care delivered.

The social determinants affect health in multiple ways, both directly and indirectly. A social determinant like air pollution affects population health directly and is demonstrated by increased rates of asthma in polluted areas, for example. Social determinants also affect health indirectly, by affecting access to coverage and care, as well as the quality of the care received—proximity to an accredited hospital, for example. All of these factors impact health outcomes.

A specific example may help. A social determinant that affects health both directly and indirectly is a low-wage and/or high-stress job with no benefits (think gig economy or working as a manicurist in a nail salon). Health is affected directly by the poor working conditions of these kinds of jobs (stress, exposure to toxins or unsafe conditions, etc.) and indirectly, by limiting the workers' access to healthcare (e.g., when the jobs don't provide health insurance). This lack of access to healthcare then impacts the ability to identify and manage chronic conditions, like diabetes, as well as be treated for acute conditions, like broken bones and heart attacks. As health deteriorates and isn't managed, job prospects diminish. It's a vicious circle.

Consider the example of Le Thi Lam, a Vietnamese immigrant who worked in a nail salon in Sacramento. She specialized in applying acrylic nails but developed a thyroid condition and asthma after three years, most likely due to the toxins in the chemicals she was using to apply the nails.

She was too sick to work, so she quit, but was unable to find another job, so returned. She developed breast cancer ten years later.[3] Or the case of Ki Ok Chung, a salon worker for close to twenty years, whose fingerprints had almost worn off due to the chemicals she worked with every day—a fact she discovered when she applied for US citizenship.[4]

Dr. Charles Hwu, an internist in Queens, New York, who serves many Asian Americans, had this to say about his patients who work for nail salons and are otherwise healthy: "They come in usually with breathing problems, some symptoms similar to an allergy, and also asthma symptoms—they cannot breathe. . . . Judging from the symptoms with these women, it seems that they are either smokers, secondhand smokers or asthma patients, but they are none of the above. They work for nail salons."[5]

"There are so many stories but no one that dares to tell them," said Nancy Otavalo, a manicurist in Queens, New York. "There are thousands of women who are working in this, but no one asking: 'What's happening to you? How do you feel?' We just work and work."[6]

I N SPITE OF THE FACT that there are so many nonmedical factors that affect health, the US has traditionally focused predominantly on *medical* care to improve individual and population health—even though inadequate medical care accounts for only 10–15 percent of preventable deaths nationwide.[7] If that sounds low to you, think about this: What impacts more Americans' health overall? Triple bypass surgeries or healthy food delivery services? Hospitalizations for pneumonia or proper ventilation in factories and office buildings? Emergency room visits for a few people or safe, affordable housing for many? Even a top neurosurgeon who performs two hundred lifesaving procedures a year can't match the impact of a public health marketer whose ad campaign cut the adolescent smoking rate by 0.1 percent. For example, a 2012 antismoking campaign that cost $54 million added 330,000 years of life to the US population.[8] That's a cost of $164 per year of life. Compare that to treating lung cancer for one person, which costs on average $46,000.[9]

Clearly, our behavior, environment, and other nonmedical circumstances have important consequences for our health. So why do Americans devote so much of our attention and resources to *medical* care, and not a broader system of social supports? I'll explore the answer to this a little later in the chapter. For now, let's look at some specific examples of the social determinants of health.

FIVE EXAMPLES OF SOCIAL DETERMINANTS

To illustrate how social determinants affect health, I've selected five representative factors for a deeper dive: education, social supports, racism, housing, and pollution. *Education* is a cornerstone of democracy and an acknowledged universal right in the US. *Social supports* are a vital aspect of strong communities and therefore population health. *Racism* drives the health disparities that exacerbate the inequities in our society and ties strongly to the social justice theme of this book. *Housing*, including location, sets the stage for physical well-being and access to key resources. And *pollution* affects all of us, regardless of our socioeconomic status.

These are all issues I have worked on throughout my life, both personally and professionally. I've learned that some are tougher to address than others: When I worked for the YWCA after college, I saw the challenges firsthand while running grassroots programs to empower women and eliminate racism on a shoestring budget. Later, as a leader in the state welfare and Medicaid programs, I encountered the complexities of working on social determinants at the political and institutional level.

EDUCATION

It's well known that education level affects job prospects, income, and social standing. What's less well known is that education level actually affects life expectancy. In fact, public health experts have stated that "for the population as a whole, the most consistent predictor of the likelihood of death in any given year is level of education."[10] Women with college or graduate degrees live an average of twelve years longer than women who didn't graduate from high school.

How does this happen? At the baseline level, education provides literacy skills and some knowledge of individual health. Remember that required course in high school that taught you about the food pyramid, safe sex, and avoiding alcohol and drug abuse? As basic as that curriculum was, it helped to level the playing field regarding fundamental health terminology and risks. But education's impact on our health goes far beyond this.

Education brings us to another level, through job opportunities, and with those jobs come income (adequate/inadequate), working conditions (safe/unsafe, healthy/unhealthy), and access to resources (health insurance/no health insurance, employee assistance programs). And finally, enough education can help bring us to a more "self-actualized" state, where we have more of a sense of control due to strong coping and problem-solving skills, as well as social networks with norms for healthy behaviors.

At the baseline level, literacy skills are critical to effectively interacting with the healthcare system, including accessing healthcare coverage. However, more than thirty million adults in the United States are unable to read, write, or do math above a third-grade level.[11] Twenty-six million people who reside in the country speak predominantly a language other than English. Low literacy adds an estimated $230 billion in healthcare costs every year.[12]

Health literacy is even more limited in the US. Polls have shown that less than 5 percent of people understand basic insurance terms, which affects people's ability to purchase insurance plans that are right for them.[13] Low health literacy is associated with increased rates of hospitalization, greater use of emergency care, reduced rates of mammography screening and influenza vaccination, and lesser ability to demonstrate taking medications appropriately and to interpret labels and health messages.[14] One study of the elderly found that those with low health literacy were half as likely to have one of three widely accepted measures of healthcare access (a regular source of medical care, an influenza vaccination within the year, or insurance for medications).[15]

Numeracy skills are another type of literacy that can affect access to healthcare coverage. Numeracy skills are influenced by education and exposure to math at home or work, as well as certain tools and your familiarity with them. One study of a large employer found that 55 percent of its employees selected a plan that was unquestionably costlier than an alternative available to them, even with the same provider network.[16] A lack of health literacy and numeracy are partially to blame, but even those well versed with health insurance often find the choices to be daunting.

Finally, patients with limited English proficiency face additional barriers to accessing healthcare—they are less likely to have a usual source of care and receive preventive services.[17] Although many providers make an effort to hire bilingual staff or provide translation services, translation services are not universally available, and a number of non-English speakers experience reduced access as a result.

SOCIAL SUPPORTS

Our social supports are among the most important factors in our health. Scientists have proven that social relationships are as powerful a factor in risk of death as smoking and alcohol, and a greater factor than physical inactivity and obesity.[18]

We live and work in a world of social connections, which includes our families, friends, and communities—their norms or established ways of doing things can range from being supportive and helpful to being hurtful. We receive different types of social feedback, both positive and negative, from our family and friends. Sometimes the feedback serves our best interests and sometimes it doesn't. Social support can inspire people to take control of their health, or to disregard it. It can provide valuable advice about interacting with the healthcare system or can lead you astray. For example, if having health insurance is uncommon in your family or community, you'll be much less likely to know how to go about obtaining it. Unfortunately, this is a life skill that isn't typically taught in a high school health class.

Research has shown the importance of strong social networks to overall health as well as the devastating impact of loneliness. Loneliness kills: People with stronger social relationships have a 50 percent increased likelihood of survival than those with weaker social relationships.[19] There's a link between low levels of social connection and depression, which in turn can result in heart attacks and cancer. The stress hormone blood profiles of socially connected people are measurably healthier than those of isolated people.[20] Social connection even affects the common cold: "In one study, researchers swabbed viruses into volunteers' noses, and the most socially connected volunteers got markedly fewer colds than the least connected."[21] To solve this, people need to connect: for folks who don't belong to any groups, joining a group will reduce risk of dying by half over the next year.[22]

I experienced the full value of social connections when I was going through my cancer diagnosis, surgery, and recovery: in addition to having support from my husband, I was fortunate to have a circle of women friends (known for twenty years as the Moms Group) and other dear friends—all like sisters to me—who surrounded me with love and comfort, accompanied me to doctors' appointments, and made sure I had the best medical advice.

Social connection and supports are even more important for people with certain health conditions, including chronic disease, mental health issues (such as depression), and disabilities. They often face daunting challenges—their conditions create barriers to accessing healthcare that can have dire consequences. For example, over a quarter of Americans who die before the age of seventy-five could have lived longer if they had received appropriate medical care for their chronic condition.[23]

One of the barriers that people with these health conditions often face is stigma. Stigma is "a perceived negative attribute that causes someone to devalue or think less of the whole person."[24] People can be stigmatized for many reasons, including their skin color, national origin, or beliefs. They can also be stigmatized for conditions like behavioral health disorders, HIV, and diabetes—many perceive the presence of these illnesses to be the fault of the afflicted. For example, the average delay for seeking help for a mood disorder in the US is eight years—nine years for anxiety disorders. This problem is compounded for people who are poorly educated or part of a racial/ethnic minority group, who are even more likely to delay seeking care.[25]

Similarly, diabetic patients sometimes do not disclose their condition to healthcare professionals out of fear of judgment.[26] Interestingly, those with type 1 diabetes, which people are born with, report higher rates of stigma than people with type 2 diabetes, which develops later in life and is caused by a combination of genetic and behavioral factors.[27] Obviously, stigma doesn't necessarily follow the lines of science or rationality.

RACISM

Racism is a social determinant with deadly consequences. As Harvard professor David Williams said so compellingly, "We have scientific evidence that discrimination is pervasive. Over 200 African-Americans die every day who would not die if they had the same health experience as whites. Think of a huge jet crashing every day—that is the kind of disparity we're talking about."[28]

It doesn't matter if the racism is intentional or unintentional.[29] If race were simply the individual-level, biological characteristic that it is, like hair or eye color, there wouldn't be racial disparities in health outcomes and other measures. But race in the US is a social construct, and racism drives these disparities. Racism can affect health coverage, as well as access to and delivery of healthcare, which ultimately affects health outcomes. For example, African Americans are less likely to have healthcare coverage or access to the healthcare system. They also face bias in the delivery of healthcare. In addition, racism has a direct effect on people's health, as numerous studies have shown regarding the effects of stress.[30] For all of these reasons, African Americans ultimately have a significantly shorter life expectancy than whites do.

Race can be correlated with differences in health outcomes both directly (physiologically, due to the stress of racism) and indirectly (lack of access to health insurance coverage limits access to healthcare, which in turn affects health outcomes).

A study in 2017 found that working-age adults from economically disadvantaged racial groups (black, Hispanic, and Native American) have lower rates of enrollment in health insurance. In fact, Hispanics and Native Americans have twice the rate of uninsurance that whites and Asian Americans do. This is partly due to differences in income, immigration status, and structural impediments to coverage. It's also a result of historical barriers that have subjugated minority groups, including the effects of racism. (See figure 7.2.)

And yet, overall life expectancy does not correlate with health insurance alone: Hispanics have a higher life expectancy than most other groups, despite their lack of health insurance coverage.[31] (See Figure 7.3.)

African Americans have lower life expectancies and higher rates of infant mortality than whites at all levels of income and educational attainment.[32] Researchers are beginning to suggest that this persistent inequality, even between highly educated and well-off African Americans and whites, can be attributed to the psychological stress of discrimination.[33]

For millions of Americans, the life-altering health consequences of certain *unchosen* personal or community circumstances can be traced back to decades of discriminatory behavior and policies. For example, the twentieth-century practice of "redlining" (the systematic denial of services and loans to minorities living in urban neighborhoods) is a policy that contributed to the

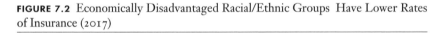

FIGURE 7.2 Economically Disadvantaged Racial/Ethnic Groups Have Lower Rates of Insurance (2017)

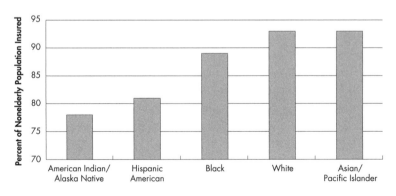

Source: "Uninsured Rates for the Nonelderly by Race/Ethnicity," Kaiser Family Foundation, last updated 2017, https://www.kff.org.

FIGURE 7.3 Economically disadvantaged racial/ethnic groups have lower life
expectancy, with some exceptions.

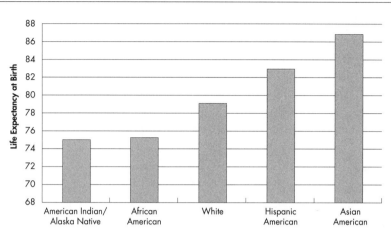

Source: WorldLifeExpectancy.com, last updated 2014, https://www.worldlifeexpectancy.com/usa/life
-expectancy-asian-american.

poverty and poor living conditions we see negatively impacting the health
of many in American cities, and those health effects have persisted, even as
redlining policies have been outlawed.

The redlining policy created a self-fulfilling prophecy for already de-
pressed urban neighborhoods, starving them of investment and ensuring
the continuation of dilapidated buildings, poor living conditions, and limited economic opportunities. In cities such as Boston, Chicago, St. Louis,
Oakland, and Atlanta, minorities were blocked from moving to other (predominantly white) neighborhoods, remaining segregated in low-resource
communities that local politicians tended to ignore. Apartments and even
schools exposed children to extensive amounts of lead in pipes and paint.

Today, little has changed. Many of the same redlined neighborhoods
have not had the investment to remove lead from buildings or provide people with access to healthy food options and safe outdoor spaces. The legacy
of slavery and history of discriminatory laws continues to translate into poor
health outcomes for African Americans today.

HOUSING AND LOCATION

The quality and location of your housing are inextricably linked to your health.
For example, extremely high and low temperatures have been associated with

increased mortality, especially among vulnerable populations such as the elderly. Injuries occurring at home result in an estimated four million emergency department visits and seventy thousand hospital admissions per year. Residential crowding is linked with tuberculosis and respiratory infections and psychological distress among both adults and children. Substandard housing conditions such as water leaks, poor ventilation, dirty carpets, and pest infestations can lead to an increase in mold, mites, and other allergens.[34] There are thirty-seven million homes in the United States with lead-based paint, and twenty-three million have at least one lead hazard. One in three homes with children younger than six has a lead-based paint hazard, with most of the exposure occurring in lower-income areas, including public housing. Lead poisoning irreversibly affects brain and nervous system development, and an estimated 310,000 children ages one to five in the US have elevated blood lead levels.

In addition to the quality of the housing itself, the location of housing also affects health. In fact, professor and public health expert Melody Goodman has said that "your ZIP code is a better predictor of your health than your genetic code."[35] Geography is a hugely important factor when it comes to having access to care. Maps from the federal government show that large geographic sections of the country are designated "medically underserved areas," regions with too few primary care doctors, or with high infant mortality rates, high levels of poverty, or large elderly populations.[36] This results in lots of people missing or not making medical appointments because they are difficult to get to. Some people who live in rural areas must travel long distances using public transit to get to appointments, increasing their likelihood of being late or not showing up. This problem is so pervasive that a number of healthcare providers have stepped in to offer transportation to their facility free of charge. Investing in an Uber ride is often more cost-efficient than wasting physician resources.

Finally, low-income neighborhoods with safety issues almost by definition have less access to resources that would help to address the social determinants of health. A Chicago-based study found that poor neighborhood safety was associated with low access to large grocery stores, pharmacies, and fitness resources.[37] Additionally, hospitals are often built in areas where potential customers have commercial insurance, and avoid places where residents are either covered by Medicaid, which pays lower rates to healthcare providers, or the uninsured, in which case they might be unable to pay for the services they receive.

POLLUTION

But man is a part of nature, and his war against nature is
inevitably a war against himself.

  —RACHEL CARSON, author of *Silent Spring*[38]

I've been an environmentalist in spirit, ever since my days of camping and backpacking as a Girl Scout. I gained an early appreciation for nature's pristine places, and was alarmed by the pollution I experienced—I can still feel the pain I felt in my lungs as a young girl from the smog that hovered over Southern California and made breathing difficult, even on a beautiful day.

Pollution comes in many forms and has enormous detrimental effects on health—far more than we may realize. Air and water quality, as well as exposure to carcinogens, lead, and tobacco, are some of the known ways pollution impacts health, including causing certain cancers. For other pollutants, researchers have an idea of the relationship but are still trying to figure out their nature. And for many conditions, including certain cancers, it is unclear if an environmental exposure causes it, or what that exposure is. In many ways, pollution is the most pervasive social determinant, since it can affect anyone, regardless of social circumstances, race, or other factors. It also compounds the effects of other social determinants, manifesting in higher rates of asthma and other chronic conditions.

The field of public health was born due to a water contamination incident in 1854. That year, London experienced a cholera outbreak that killed hundreds of people. The belief at the time was that airborne particles called "miasmata" were responsible for making people sick. A physician named John Snow proposed an alternate theory, suggesting that the illness was caused by water, and he walked around the neighborhood of the outbreak knocking on doors, eventually figuring out that those who had fallen ill had all used the same water pump. In the first dramatic act of public health intervention, Dr. Snow tore the handle from the pump, rendering it useless and the people of the neighborhood safe.

Experts in environmental health have built on John Snow's work and helped uncover a number of pollutants and their effects on health. But even though we know about these harmful relationships, millions of Americans are still subject to these exposures. Only a few years ago, as many as a hundred thousand residents of Flint, Michigan, were exposed to dangerous levels of lead in their drinking water, potentially causing irreversible damage to the developing brains of some eight thousand children.[39] Although a federal state of emergency was declared in 2016, the remedies to what became known as the Flint water crisis are ongoing and leave many doubting if the water is safe to drink even today.[40]

The links between exposure and health outcomes can be difficult to pinpoint. First, researchers must separate the "culprit" exposure from all the other exposures people have in their daily lives. Additionally, many industries have vested interests in keeping their products free from regulation and have fought hard to keep their products in the market, as the pesticides industry did in initially preventing the banning of DDT in the 1970s and as the tobacco industry did when it wanted to continue to claim in marketing materials that cigarettes were healthy.[41] More recently, the cosmetics industry fought back hard and won when a coalition of nail salon workers tried to get California to restrict the use of toxic chemicals in salons. And yet, according to the Environmental Protection Agency (EPA), seventeen of the twenty common nail product ingredients that cause health problems are hazardous to the respiratory tract. In the EPA's nail salon worker safety brochure, a typical citation for a nail product ingredient states that "overexposure may cause irritation to eyes, skin, and respiratory tract" and mentions other, asthma-like symptoms, such as labored breathing and shortness of breath; it also points out that some ingredients may cause more serious side effects, including liver, kidney, and reproductive system harm.[42]

THE INTERACTION EFFECT

The social determinants of health don't operate in isolation—they are interwoven, and their interaction impacts health. Employment is a good example of this, as shown in figure 7.4. Social determinants affect the type of job you get, which in turn affects your health through a combination of factors: working conditions, work-related resources (like access to health insurance), and income.

Taking this one level deeper, it is possible to zero in on the aspect of work that directly relates to health coverage: the availability of employer-sponsored insurance. Remember, Americans rely heavily on employers for health insurance, even though only about half of employers offer health insurance to their employees. If an employer doesn't offer coverage, employees are left to purchase health insurance on their own, in the individual market. This takes a large bite out of take-home pay and is unaffordable for many people; 13 percent of *employed* people are uninsured.

FIGURE 7.4 Social context, educational attainment, and racism affect each other and have an impact on employment, which in turn affects health.

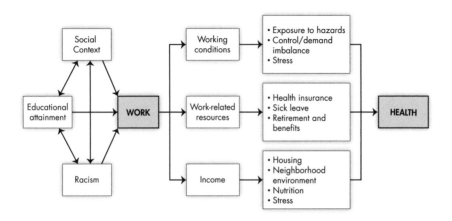

Source: Day Health Strategies, as informed by Education Matters for Health. *Robert Wood Johnson Foundation Commission to Build a Healthier America*. Issue Brief 6: Education and Health, Sept. 2009. http://www .commissiononhealth.org/PDF/c270deb3-ba42-4fbd-baeb-2cd65956f00e/Issue%20Brief%206%20Sept %2009%20-%20Education%20and%20Health.pdf.

However, being unemployed is a worse situation—unemployed people are three times as likely to be uninsured as employed people are. Over one-third of unemployed people are uninsured, and uninsured people are much more likely to delay or forgo needed care because of cost.

Taking this a step further, employer-sponsored insurance access (or lack thereof) can also be tied back to racism. Racism is a social determinant that affects employment opportunities and hiring patterns due to both histori-cal legacy and current discrimination. One result can be seen in figure 7.5: the percentage of people with employer-sponsored insurance varies signifi-cantly by race, with Asian Americans and whites being much more likely to have employer-sponsored coverage than are blacks, Hispanics, or Native Americans.

The effect of this racial disparity in health insurance coverage com-pounds, since the type of insurance people have critically affects their access to healthcare. Those with commercial health insurance (usually employer-sponsored) typically fare the best, with few limitations on access to health-care providers. By contrast, people with Medicaid coverage have less access to healthcare providers since many providers limit the numbers of Medicaid

FIGURE 7.5 Economically disadvantaged racial/ethnic groups have lower rates of employer-sponsored insurance.

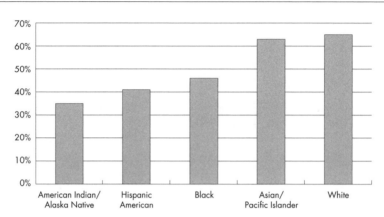

Source: "Employer-Sponsored Coverage Rates for the Nonelderly by Race/Ethnicity," Kaiser Family Foundation, https://www.kff.org.

patients they will see.[43] Furthermore, some Medicaid patients report being treated dismissively by providers.

That said, Medicaid does perform comparably or even better than commercial coverage when it comes to a number of standard measures of healthcare access, as shown in the figure 7.6. And, as the value of employer-sponsored insurance erodes for millions of people, the benefits of the Medicaid program look better and better. This is fueling some of the current "Medicaid for More" proposals that I will describe in chapter 10. It is abundantly clear that having decent health insurance is better than being uncovered.

A reminder: decent health insurance is publicly subsidized, whether through employers or through Medicaid. Because employer-sponsored health insurance is not taxed, the federal government forgoes $250 billion of revenue each year to support this benefit. This huge subsidy for taxpayers predominantly benefits the middle class, and therefore disproportionately benefits white people. As I will explain in chapter 11, there are other, and potentially better, ways some of this money could be spent.

One final note: the effects of social determinants are amplified for people with certain health conditions. For example, people with disabilities face discrimination, even though it is illegal under United States law.[44] However, people's job prospects are still affected: an employer can legally *not*

FIGURE 7.6 Adults with commercial or medicaid health plan coverage have better access to care and are more likely to receive preventive care services than uninsured adults.

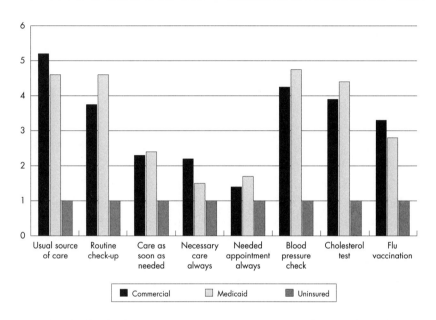

Source: "The Value of Medicaid: Access to Care and Preventive Care Services," AHIP, last modified April 9, 2018, https://www.ahip.org/the-value-of-medicaid-access-to-care-and-preventive-care-services.

hire someone based on their disability if that disability substantially affects their ability to perform the core job functions, or if accommodating the disability would cause significant difficulty or expense. The unemployment rate for disabled people was 10.7 percent in 2015, compared to 5.1 percent for nondisabled people.[45]

RISING INEQUALITY

An issue that contributes to and exacerbates the effects of social determinants is economic inequality. Economic inequality (both wealth and income) is growing at an astounding rate and has hit crisis levels in the US. It poses a serious threat to our society for many reasons. Chief among them is that inequality is bad for our collective health. As political scientist James Morone says, "Great differences in wealth . . . create great differences in health."[46]

At a recent screening of a documentary on how the opioid crisis is affecting my neighborhood in Somerville, I was struck by the feelings of inadequacy many longtime residents were expressing in the face of rising gentrification. Many are turning to opioids for relief. Studies show that falling behind economically causes stress and illness, including depression and hypertension, which leads to higher death rates.[47]

What's happening in Somerville is happening across the country. In fact, inequality in the US is at close to an all-time high.[48] In 2016, the richest 0.1 percent of Americans (think Warren Buffett, Bill Gates, Jeff Bezos) owned almost as much wealth as *everyone* in the bottom 90 percent.[49] Another example: the top twenty-five fund managers in the US make more money than all of the kindergarten teachers in the US, combined.[50] Similarly, Jeff Bezos of Amazon makes more money in one minute than the median American worker makes in one year. Since the early 1970s, the pay for average American workers has not increased, even though the economy has more than tripled in size. Most of the income gains have gone to those at the top.

International comparisons make this even more stark. In 1970, inequality in the US was close to the levels of other wealthy nations like Germany and Sweden, but by 2010, inequality in the US was much closer to that of developing nations, like Mexico and Brazil.[51] Globalization is a culprit—it's widening the gap between rich and poor in many countries. However, during that same forty-year period, most wealthy countries enacted policies such as cash transfers and social supports to reduce income disparities. As a result, despite globalization's harmful impacts, these countries are actually *more equal* today than they were a generation ago. In contrast, the US cut taxes and only modestly increased social supports, and inequality grew.

And it gets worse. Despite our beliefs, the US actually has a lower degree of social mobility than European countries do.[52] Let that sink in. We see ourselves as the land of equal opportunity, spurred on by upwardly mobile immigrants. And yet many wealthy people (an estimated 35–45 percent) actually inherited their wealth.[53]

Studies show that people live longer when they live in more egalitarian settings. As Harvard School of Public Health professor Ichiro Kawachi writes, "Health is an exquisitely sensitive mirror of our social conditions and political arrangements."[54] There's a psychological stress of inequality that affects people up and down the income spectrum.[55] The more inequality there is, the less healthy people are: inequality is correlated with higher rates of depression, hypertension, smoking, teen pregnancy, and lower self-rated health. "Living in an unequal society is toxic to just about everybody's health, and our poor ranking against other economically advanced countries can't simply be blamed on the misbehaving minority at the tail end of the bell curve," Kawachi concludes.[56]

INVESTMENT IN MEDICAL CARE VERSUS SOCIAL SERVICES

Despite the knowledge about the impact of social determinants and rising inequality on health, there is a huge disconnect in the US between healthcare and social services (nonmedical interventions and supports) that could address these issues. This occurs for many reasons. Historically, our social services and healthcare systems developed in a bifurcated way, unlike what happened in other countries. There was traditionally a lack of government involvement in social services in the US—those needs were addressed more through community-based organizations funded by voluntary contributions. Elizabeth Bradley and Lauren Taylor summed it up in their excellent book *The American Health Care Paradox*: "American reliance on voluntary organizations to meet community needs became well established by the mid-1800s, supported by traditional American values, such as individualism, hostility to centralized power, and separation of church and state."[57] Contrast this with medical care, which began getting more national attention and government investment during and immediately after World War II. By then the path was set, and the dichotomy persists to our present day.

And yet it's well documented that social service programs have a positive impact on health. There is plenty of research showing that health outcomes are more closely aligned with social service spending than with health spending.[58] As Bradley and Taylor note, "The role social services can play in preventing illnesses, mitigating repeat occurrences, or helping people manage chronic health conditions, is appreciated but underutilized, according to care providers, clients, and patients."[59] Furthermore, "Providers throughout the health care arena know that the impact of their work is being diluted by the chasm between health and social services."

There are ways to change this. Despite our nation's reluctance to invest public funds in social programs, some innovative leaders have gone ahead and built effective programs locally to address social determinants. Some are implementing new types of contracts for healthcare providers that reward health outcomes rather than health services. Known as paying for "value, not volume," these types of contracts are expected to overtake traditional fee-for-service contracts within a few years. Efforts in this area are growing in size and number and they deserve our support.

And there are many other grassroots solutions. We can take a social determinants approach to healthcare access by continuing to fund navigator programs that help people find and use their health coverage appropriately. And we must invest in community health centers, many of which were established in the 1960s, and approach healthcare holistically, the same way Mississippi's Delta Health Center (described in chapter 3) does. "[Community health centers] have strong understandings and experienced approaches to social determinants. They are well-versed in identifying problems like poor nutrition, homelessness, joblessness, dangerous or unhealthy social situations, and unhealthy environmental exposures. These centers run or have relationships with community-based organizations running programs which address these problems, and frequently refer their patients to these resources."[60] These organizations are typically nonprofits and welcome donations and volunteer support.

Some social determinants programs are showing a great return on investment. For example, the Montefiore Health System in the Bronx is addressing the housing crisis in its area by investing in twenty housing units for its chronically ill patients, as well as in respite facilities for temporary stays. Montefiore was experiencing lots of utilization of its emergency department by homeless and chronically ill people. Many of the patients they referred to shelters ended up returning to the hospital, which was not an effective way to care for the patient, cost the health system money, and took up beds that might be needed by other patients. Giving Montefiore's patients a place to stay at night not only prevented unnecessary utilization, but also returned 300 percent on the investment.[61]

Somerville, where I live, took a big step in the right direction with its Shape Up Somerville campaign, launched in 2002. The mayor, school superintendent, and numerous community-based organizations banded together to tackle childhood obesity through a series of initiatives, both in and outside of school. From healthier food in school cafeterias, to farm stands in low-income housing areas, to citywide "Let's Move" activities, the commitment was deep and far-reaching, and the activities were fun and innovative. My children benefited from this holistic approach, as did their classmates, who may not have had the same messages and opportunities at home. And the results showed: Somerville reduced childhood obesity.[62]

. . .

O THER WEALTHY COUNTRIES' GOVERNMENTS invest more in social ser-vices than the US government does. The results: their life expectancy improves while they devote fewer resources to healthcare, whereas life expectancy in the US falls further behind with each passing year.

And these results impact *all* Americans: Studies have shown that upper-income white Americans who are insured and college-educated are less healthy than their peers in other wealthy countries.[63] There are many reasons for this, including the lack of focus on preventive healthcare, and the lack of a social safety net. Job loss is particularly hard on Americans at all income levels, due to the relatively lower value of income protections in the US as compared to other developed countries.[64] Also, when Americans lose their jobs, they often lose their health coverage at the same time, which adds another devastating blow—the combined stress can trigger depression and poor health.

Given all of this evidence, why does this bifurcation between medical care and social services persist in the US? It has largely been driven by financial factors. Healthcare providers are paid to *treat* illness rather than to *prevent* it. Another factor has been the profitability of the healthcare market. As Bradley and Taylor say, "Spurred by private sector confidence in a growing and profitable health care market, the US has favored investments in health care over social services."[65] In effect, we are allowing people to get sick so the health system can profit by making them better.

Another reason for the disconnect: optics. When a health system saves (or fails to save) someone from an emergency, it's visible. In contrast, no one notices when emergencies and other health issues are prevented. Prevention is simply less exciting, despite being incredibly effective. You won't find a headline that reads "Rosemarie Day's Diabetes Is Well Managed and Under Control." On the medical side, there's a prevention brand of medicine that values caring for the whole person, understanding their needs over time, and monitoring and preventing emergencies. It's called *incrementalism*. Unfortunately, it isn't as well resourced as traditional fee-for-service medical care, and the causal link to improved outcomes is less apparent, even if more potent. On the social services and public health side, solutions like providing more healthy foods to underserved neighborhoods have proven to be challenging to implement. Combine this with the fact that we don't have enough links between traditional medicine and social services, and a picture begins to emerge of reasons prevention doesn't get enough attention. Also, people typically don't march in the streets to increase payments for primary care or social service providers.

Lastly, the people who would most benefit from public health and social service programs tend to be less powerful. For example, people with substance use disorders or poorly managed chronic conditions have often (but not always) been lower income and without the resources and connections that help move the political needle. This is changing with the opioid epidemic, which has brought these issues squarely into the hearts and homes of middle-class families.

The upshot, explained by Bradley and Taylor, is that "the health care sector bears the brunt of an inadequate social service sector."[66] Put another way, healthcare providers get the downstream effects of inadequate investments made upstream.

If we want to improve our nation's health, then taking a broader, more holistic view of what affects health is key. So is having a sense of shared responsibility for our larger community, and not thinking about poor health as based entirely on "individual choices and failings."[67] We need to push for solutions beyond health insurance coverage, and beyond the healthcare system itself. Shape Up Somerville provides a great example of this, as a community-based, public health approach to tackling childhood obesity.

Understanding initiatives like these can help us to be better informed activists. Programs that address the social determinants of health enhance people's productivity and can save money in the long run. Everyone benefits. Funds could be freed up from health spending and used for other programs such as education or workforce investments. With these investments, the US labor force would become more robust, strengthened by a society that helps develop talent instead of just focusing on one health emergency after the next. With better jobs, people could have more income to spend, which in turn circulates through the economy and leads to even more jobs and successful businesses. And there could be less crime and social strife because more people live better and happier lives.

The social determinants of health are systemic in nature and, as with making healthcare a right, will require collective action and political intervention to address. The stakes are high—failing to invest in them will cause our economy to perform less well and will result in more disparity, poverty, and sickness for all Americans. It's time to urge the healthcare system and public policymakers to pay more attention to the social determinants of health.

CHAPTER 8

SOLUTIONS NEED TO BE POLITICAL, NOT POLARIZING

To the extent that it is possible . . . you must live in the world today as you wish everyone to live in the world to come. That can be your contribution. Otherwise, the world you want will never be formed. Why? Because you are waiting for others to do what you are not doing; and they are waiting for you, and so on.

—ALICE WALKER, *Temple of My Familiar*[1]

IN MY JOB AS A HEALTHCARE CONSULTANT, I often talk with women (and men) about how politics affects our healthcare system. I might spend the morning discussing federal health reform proposals with a state exchange leader and the afternoon explaining the risks of new health insurance models to a hospital CEO. But outside of work, most women I know don't want to engage in those kinds of conversations. Why? One reason is that they may worry they don't know enough about the subject. Another is that they think healthcare has become "too political." They don't want to inadvertently say something offensive or get drawn into a potentially contentious debate that ends up being more about politicians than policy.

But what are women risking by shying away from conversations about healthcare, even if those conversations *do* relate to politics? To answer that question, let me explain how US healthcare and politics are intertwined, starting at the individual, or personal, level.

THE PERSONAL IS POLITICAL

Many political issues are based on what people care about personally. But what is it that gets us to care deeply enough about a personal issue that we connect to it politically? Studies show that, when it comes to political issues, there are three main drivers: our own self-interest, empathy for others, and our values.[2] Regardless of the source of our connection to an issue, once we care about it, we tend to stay focused on it, even when other political issues heat up. We devote attention to the issue. We stay informed. We think about it and talk about it. We also remember the issue better than other competing issues, and it tends to bring on stronger emotions.

In other words, "The personal is political." This is a phrase that was popularized by feminists, including Gloria Steinem, in the 1960s and 1970s. It's been interpreted in many ways since then, but in an early piece about the value of consciousness-raising groups, essayist Carol Hanisch explained that so-called personal issues such as childcare and the division of household labor, are, in fact, political. She says:

> One of the first things we discover in these groups is that *personal problems are political problems.* There are no personal solutions at this time. *There is only collective action for a collective solution.*[3] (Emphasis mine.)

Healthcare consumer decisions are personal and are made primarily by women (at the household level). But when those decisions are impeded by significant systemic roadblocks, such as health insurance market failures and a lack of access to healthcare coverage, the personal must evolve, and a political solution is needed.

If you're like many people, you probably have strongly held views regarding access to healthcare. These views are shaped by your personal situation and your values. If you or someone you love is very ill or has a chronic condition, then access to healthcare is a particularly salient issue for you. More generally, you may value access to healthcare due to a general belief in social justice, or a specific belief in healthcare as a right.

The strength of your feelings about healthcare coverage may vary over time, depending on your situation, or the situation of those you love. Personally, my commitment to universal healthcare has always been rooted in my strong belief in social justice. My empathy and commitment are even deeper now, due to the reality of my cancer diagnosis. Even though my cancer was successfully treated, I now have a permanent preexisting condition—and I have joined the millions of others who, without the ACA's protections, face the same potential barriers to healthcare access. These barriers are systemic and can't be solved by any one of us at the individual level. They are so large and important that they cry out for a national, political solution similar to what was accomplished with Medicare, Medicaid, and the ACA. But those measures didn't go far enough—we need universal healthcare.

The challenge is that universal healthcare is an issue of national importance, but issues of personal importance are bigger drivers of our political behavior. Studies show that "when evaluating candidates for public office, making vote choices, and expressing policy preferences directly to elected officials and the news media, *citizens are focused primarily on policy issues they consider to be personally important* rather than issues they consider to be nationally important."[4] (Emphasis mine.)

So, what steps can we take to move healthcare access from being personally important to being addressed at the national level? First, people who care about healthcare access as a personal issue need to share their stories and make their feelings known, collectively, to the media and "the powers that be." Many women already feel strongly about their frustrations and worries about healthcare coverage, but they may not be aware that lots of people feel the same way. Some women may not yet feel strongly, but once they hear other people's stories about the healthcare system, a form of "radical empathy" develops. With this heightened awareness, and empathy for others, people may develop "enlightened preferences"—preferences that go beyond their immediate self-interest.[5] I believe that building this kind of collective awareness is the key to women having the energy, strength, and numbers to influence the democratic process around national healthcare reform.

In a democracy, there is typically a great deal of deliberation around what our government does. As citizens, we can influence that process by whom we elect and by the donations we make, and by the other ways we "show up." We can also bring attention to universal healthcare by "agenda setting," i.e., getting the media to focus on it (through events, op-eds, and more). All of these activities are considered "getting political," in a principled sort of way. I'll explain more about how to engage politically and use the power of collective action in chapter 12.

Of course, we can't ignore the fact that there are powerful corporate and stakeholder groups (such as hospitals, doctors, and insurers) who influence the political process through lobbying, campaign contributions, and more. But grassroots groups of women can also organize to launch and support candidates, make donations, get the media's attention, and stay informed. And at the end of the day, it's the votes that count. The bottom line is that women can drive change by getting political and voting in large numbers on priority issues like universal healthcare.

POLITICS AT THE NATIONAL LEVEL

Unfortunately, many women are uncomfortable with how polarized politics has become. They see Democrats and Republicans staying in their respective camps, without much overlap in policy priorities.[6] A lot of women would prefer to find some common ground on the issues, rather than engage in heated debates.

It's an understandable concern. Congress is measurably more polarized than it was in the 1970s. As a result, Congress is passing fewer laws than it used to.[7] At first glance, it's hard to say which became polarized first: the electorate or Congress. There are so many factors in play. But digging more deeply, political scientists have shown that the electorate isn't any more polarized than it was before the civil rights movement. Instead the electorate has "sorted" itself into political parties in a more consistent way (for example, conservative Southern whites who used to be Democrats are now Republicans, and the Northeast, which once had a large number of moderate Republicans, now has more Democrats due to the shift in demographics resulting from urbanization and immigration).

When it comes to Congress, however, it turns out that Republicans have moved further to the right than Democrats have moved to the left.[8] Nolan McCarty, a political scientist who has studied political polarization, states,

> Despite the widespread belief that both parties have moved to the extremes, the movement of the Republican Party to the right accounts for most of the divergence between the two parties. Since the 1970s, each new cohort of Republican legislators has taken [more] conservative positions on legislation than the cohorts before them. That is not true of Democratic legislators.[9]

This is known as "asymmetric polarization," and political scientists Thomas Mann and Norman Ornstein believe that it is the main reason for our current political dysfunction. In their words: "When one party moves this far from the mainstream, it makes it nearly impossible for the political system to deal constructively with the country's challenges."[10] I would call this "dysfunctional polarization."

As the parties have become more polarized, there has been a large and growing number of independents—people in the political middle who don't affiliate with a political party. There were more registered independent voters (37 percent) than either Democrats (33 percent) or Republicans (26 percent) in 2017.[11] The share of independent voters has grown since 1994 (from

30 percent to 37 percent). While most independents lean toward one party or another, they will cross party lines when they vote, which opens up opportunities for gaining their support for universal healthcare. Turning back to healthcare, we can see that the ACA has been a living example of the dysfunctional polarization described above. The debate leading up to the passage of the ACA in 2010, and the ensuing years that culminated in the "repeal and replace" efforts of 2017, has been very politically polarized. Contrary to what many believe, however, the ACA did not cause this polarization. As discussed above, it was already there.[12]

A movement for universal healthcare needs to be understood in this context. Since the polarized environment is a given, is it possible to find a path forward? As I look back over what I learned about the politics around the ACA, I can see strategies that could apply toward a movement for universal healthcare. They include understanding the reasons for opposition to the ACA.

In chapter 2, I summarized the path that Democrats took to pass the ACA. The Democrats managed to enact the ACA in a polarized environment, in which bipartisan common ground was hard to come by. They attempted a bipartisan solution, but in the end, as in the passage of Medicaid and Medicare in 1965, they were able to pass the law because there were Democratic majorities in Congress and a Democratic president. Unfortunately, a good deal of ACA opposition stemmed from an opportunistic form of politics, intended to score political points, rather than address issues. This political opposition fueled the large and vociferous number of ACA repeal attempts, which stoked the polarized environment even more, making it difficult to find compromise. Since many elected Republicans have moved further to the right, it's hard to imagine them proposing a Nixon or Bush type of healthcare coverage program, even a partial one, in the current environment. Interestingly, Democrats incorporated many Republican ideas in the ACA, including its market-based solutions. Despite that, Republicans have remained opposed to the ACA. Why?

One category of opposition is *values-based*: there are several fundamental values-based differences of opinion that people may have about the core tenets of the ACA. The first is that government's role should be limited and not interfere in the private market or in regulating people's lives. Libertarians and others believe that government shouldn't require people to pay for things they don't want. The opposition to the individual mandate is wrapped up in this ideology, although conservative opposition to the individual mandate, based on values or something else, was not visible until President Barack Obama embraced it in 2009. Others, including about 30 percent of Republicans, do not believe that healthcare is a right. This ties to their view that government's role should be limited (since it's the government that would be charged with enforcing the right).

Another category of opposition involves *individual fairness*, i.e., how people believe their personal situation compares to that of others. Focus groups have shown that people who qualify for subsidized healthcare through the ACA believe they should get it for free, if they see that others are. There are conservatives, including Trump supporters needing health insurance, who resent the fact that some people get free Medicaid coverage, while they themselves have to pay something through Healthcare.gov.[13] Related to this is the notion that people shouldn't be "getting something for nothing." Resentment builds in multiple ways.

In the same vein, there are those who feel that it's unfair that they must pay more for insurance than they did before the ACA. This has been exacerbated by the rising cost of premiums. The fact is, healthy people in the individual insurance market do have to pay more than they'd had to if they bought insurance before the ACA. That said, the insurance now covers more benefits and guarantees coverage when people get sick. What healthy people may not see are the trade-offs: sicker people are no longer shut out of buying insurance, and no one knows what the future holds in terms of their own health.

Beyond the values-based and individual fairness differences, I believe there was another underlying current of opposition to the ACA: a repugnant opposition rooted in racism and dislike of President Obama. Some people, from Senator Mitch McConnell on down, were anti-Obama, no matter what the issue. The label "Obamacare" was popularized by conservative opponents to the law, not by advocates. Since the online marketplaces were strongly identified with President Obama, some people stayed away. The connection of this public resource to our former president has politicized it much more than similar government-run services, like Medicaid.

Finally, some of the opposition to the ACA was ostensibly based on the ACA's costs (which opponents claimed would increase the federal deficit), as well as the new taxes built into the ACA. (The concern about the size of the deficit was also folded into Republican proposals to replace the ACA by curtailing spending through block granting the Medicaid program.) The new costs of the ACA were actually paid for through a combination of healthcare taxes and program savings. Instead, it is the Tax Cuts Act of 2017 (which re-pealed the individual mandate penalty) that will increase the federal deficit. But the fact that new taxes were included in the ACA may have been the "third rail" for many Republicans. This opens a discussion on deciding what our societal priorities should be, in terms of taxing and spending, which I'll address in chapter 11. It's important to understand the opposition to the ACA. But we don't have to get bogged down by the disagreement and ob-structionism. Yes, the issue is political, and the environment is polarized, but it is possible to overcome these obstacles and move forward with enacting universal healthcare.

In chapter 2, I explained that at several key moments in our history, the opposition to healthcare expansion has been overcome. Early calls for coverage expansion, including for Medicare and Medicaid, elicited concerns about "socialized medicine" (a.k.a. government-controlled healthcare). This concern about the extent of government's role is a common theme through-out our history, and it was shared by many in the healthcare establishment, including doctors and hospital executives who were concerned about gov-ernment controlling their reimbursements or setting their pay.

Yet, despite these politics, "the arc of health policy continues to bend toward increasing coverage."[14] Here are some things that I find particularly interesting about the history of expanded healthcare coverage in the US that point the way to strategies to enact universal healthcare.

First, conservatives supported expanding healthcare coverage up until very recently. They offered many proposals and counterproposals, and many of their ideas were incorporated in Democrats' solutions, including the ACA. And conservatives now support Medicare, which has made the status of the elderly far more equal than any other segment of our society.

Second, when universal coverage couldn't happen, incremental changes were often made instead, such as establishment of the Children's Health Insurance Program. These often happened in a bipartisan way.

Third, federal legislators have worked around political conundrums by allowing states to opt into a program, or choose their solution, rather than imposing a national one (this has been especially true for Medicaid). It takes a while, but states eventually join in—similar to the original rollout of the Medicaid program, we are seeing this happen again with the ACA's "Medic-aid expansion" opportunity, where, little by little, more states are opting in.

Fourth, once programs like Medicare and Medicaid are implemented, they "stick." People get used to having the comfort of additional healthcare coverage for themselves or their family members. Then the issue becomes how to keep funding them. As I'll discuss in chapter 11, finding the funding for universal coverage is possible—it's about priorities.

Finally, persistent public pressure works. Medicare was enacted thanks to strong activism, and the ACA has not (yet) been repealed because of the public outcry and the pressure that activists from organizations like Moms-Rising put on politicians.

These lessons from our coverage expansion history give us some potential stepping-stones for a path forward. But above all, this simple fact remains: the fundamental currency of politics is votes. With enough women's votes, the opposition to universal healthcare can be overcome.

HEALTHCARE AND WOMEN'S VOTES

The good news is that healthcare is a critical issue to most voters. In fact, it ranked as the top issue for voters in the 2018 midterm elections,[15] and was an "extremely important issue" for voters in the 2016 presidential election, when it was the first priority for Democrats and fourth for independents and Republicans.[16] But it is even more important to women across the political spectrum. In 2016, 41 percent of female voters said that healthcare was "extremely important" to their vote whereas only 31 percent of male voters said that it was extremely important.[17]

There's a long-standing gender gap in voter affiliation: women are more likely to identify as Democrats or lean toward the Democratic Party than men are. This gap has grown in recent years, as more women are leaning Democratic (56 percent of women versus 44 percent of men in 2017, compared with 48 percent of women and 39 percent of men in 1994).[18] The gender gap may be explained by the fact that Democratic candidates tend to campaign on things like expanding social and worker supports, such as healthcare and increasing the minimum wage.[19] Notably, this strong support for Democrats among women is due in large part to African American women, who lean heavily Democratic. In the 2018 election, black women voted for Democrats 92 percent of the time, whereas only 49 percent of white women voted for Democrats.

The gender gap persists when you drill down into more specific questions about healthcare. For example, when asked, "How important is it to you that health insurance be affordable for all Americans?," 87 percent of female respondents said it was "very important," but only 75 percent of men did. The gap in political party was even greater: 95 percent of Democrats said it was "very important" whereas only 64 percent of Republicans did.[20]

However, it's important to note that women are divided by political party affiliation in their actual healthcare priorities. For example, more Democratic than Republican women voters supported increasing access to healthcare (31 percent versus 14 percent) in 2016 while at the same time Republican women supported a repeal of the ACA in greater numbers. One area of common ground for women across party lines is making healthcare more affordable. This suggests that any universal healthcare initiative should address healthcare affordability for all, to have broader acceptance.

Once women start engaging in collective action around universal healthcare, we can create a social movement that sets the agenda in the political arena through culture change (via the stories we share and the media attention we get) and ultimately, our votes. After all, in a democracy, power is conferred on elected officials by votes. It's as simple as that. Politicians must be elected to have power. Yes, financial contributions matter; politicians need resources to get their word out during campaigns. But at the end of the day, it boils down to whether they can get the votes. As Cecile Richards said,

> Now more than ever, women are the most important political force in America. We have enormous power to change the direction of this country, and it's time to use it. Marching, knitting and protesting are great. But voting, and changing who is elected to office, is essential.[21]

Every single one of us can vote, and when those votes are organized across hundreds or thousands or millions of people—and are focused on a desired outcome like healthcare for all—they are even more powerful. Remember: every vote counts. It is not unusual for elections to be decided by just a few votes. The 2000 presidential election (Bush versus Gore) was decided by only 537 votes in Florida. Women are already voting at higher rates than men. In the 2016 presidential election, of the 139 million people who voted, 74 million (54 percent) were women and 64 million (46 percent) were men. But there were still plenty of women who didn't vote. There are some 116 million women who are eligible to vote, but in 2016, only 84 million women were registered to do so. Then, just 74 million of them actually voted. Add together the 32 million unregistered women and the 10 million registered, but nonvoting women, and that's 42 million missing votes from women!

Another resource that hasn't been fully tapped is the *independent* vote. We tend to think about healthcare voters in relation to Democratic or Republican Party candidates and platforms. But when looking to turn out potential and actual voters, it's important to remember that most voters don't affiliate with a party, and it's a growing number of people. While this growth has been driven more by men than by women, independent women voters lean Democratic when they vote (56 percent voted Democratic in 2018 compared to 51 percent of men),[22] making them good targets for a universal health coverage message. Independent voters are key to swaying the presidential election and certain Senate races—they hold a lot of power if they make universal healthcare their top priority.

Finally, the unrealized potential of these untapped votes (women who didn't vote and independents who vote and can sway outcomes) is underscored by polling data that shows support for universal healthcare has risen over the past four years: 60 percent of people now say that "it is the responsibility of the federal government to ensure that all Americans have health coverage," up from 42 percent in 2013.[23]

THERE IS NO WAY TO AVOID the politics of making access to healthcare universal. And the reality is that our current politics are polarized. But we can find a workable path if we tap into women's need for a solution. We must take the personal and make it political. Women are united through caregiving pressures, family responsibilities, and concerns about affordable healthcare. If we tap into this collective stress and pain, we can build passion for the cause of universal healthcare.

At the same time, we must be pragmatic. We live in a country that strongly values individual freedom and distrusts government solutions. These values were present in the ACA debate and underlie our polarized politics. As I've traveled the country to help implement health reform, I've worked in a diverse array of states, from Hawaii, to Montana, to Kentucky, to Rhode Island. I have worked with insurers and state officials. I have seen that we cannot change everyone's minds—some values are too strongly held. But we can find a workable solution. To truly bridge the gap between the values of individual freedom and the ideal of universal healthcare, we must tread carefully and find balanced solutions. There's an opportunity to tap into a large group of people, including independent voters, who dislike the political extremes and would like to see practical solutions to our healthcare problems.

When I was a graduate student, Professor Mary Jo Bane at the Harvard Kennedy School made a big impression on me when she talked about finding the balance between having "hard heads and soft hearts"—she meant for us to be analytical and seek fact-based policy solutions, while at the same time maintaining our empathy for real people and their situations.

There are many possibilities for empathetic, yet fact-based policy solutions and the paths they offer to universal healthcare. I'll explore several of these in the next few chapters, and as you read on, keep the lessons of history in mind, as well as the understanding about values that emerged in the ACA debates.

I opened the chapter with this thought: "You must live in the world today as you wish everyone to live in the world to come." Let's dwell in that possibility.

CHAPTER 9

■ ■ ■ ■ ■ ■

OTHER COUNTRIES LEAD THE WAY

The development of a society, rich or poor, can be judged by the quality of its population's health, how fairly health is distributed across the social spectrum, and the degree of protection provided from disadvantage as a result of ill-health.

—WORLD HEALTH ORGANIZATION[1]

Duration my adult life, I have had the good fortune to travel internationally, and through these experiences, I've found lots to admire about other cultures. That's always left me curious about why some Americans seem so reluctant to learn from other countries—particularly if these countries have found answers to problems we are still struggling to solve.

T. R. Reid, who wrote *The Healing of America* and greatly influenced my thinking about healthcare systems in other countries, sums it up beautifully when he says, "The real patriot, the person who genuinely loves his country, or college, or company, is the person who recognizes problems and tries to fix them."[2] I couldn't agree more. And with that in mind, consider this:

The United States is the only developed country that does not have universal healthcare. Let that sink in for a minute. The *only* developed country.

And what's more, our population's health outcomes are much worse than those of countries that have universal healthcare, despite the tremendous amount we spend. In fact, our infant mortality and life expectancy rates are similar to those of much poorer nations. American women are much more likely to die in pregnancy and childbirth than they are in any other wealthy country (with black women three to four times more likely to die than white women), and the rate is getting worse.[3] American women have higher rates of emotional distress and are the least likely to give a high rating to the quality of their healthcare, compared to women in other wealthy countries. And almost half of American women have problems with their medical bills.

Which raises this big question: how is it that we are exceptional in so many of our healthcare achievements, including the lifesaving advances we've made through cutting-edge science and technology, but are failing in these most basic ways? For a country that prides itself on being the best, how can we let other countries surpass us with regard to something as fundamental as our health? And for a country that loves making smart investments through capitalism, how can we tolerate such a low return on investment?

To begin answering these questions, let's take a look at how other countries achieve better outcomes.

MAKING HEALTHCARE UNIVERSAL

Every developed country has wrestled with the challenge of how to ensure the health of its citizens. Those who have succeeded have at least one thing in common: they provide universal coverage. Their motivations vary, from moral to political to economic. The way they provide universal coverage also varies (tremendously): they range from Britain's single-payer system to Germany's multipayer system. To provide a representative sample of these different approaches, I looked at over a dozen countries, including Australia, Canada, Denmark, France, Germany, Britain, the Netherlands, Sweden, Switzerland, Singapore, and Taiwan. Ultimately, I chose three: Britain, Canada, and Germany. Let's dive in.

BRITAIN

We cover everybody, but we don't cover everything.

    —JOHN REID, British health minister[4]

Britain's healthcare system, the National Health Service (NHS), is one of the most well-known health systems in the world. It is both a *single-payer* and a (mostly) *government provider* system.[5] Nine out of ten people in Britain receive all of their healthcare through the NHS.[6] Private coverage options are available but are not widely used.

Britain's healthcare system was conceived of during the final days of World War II, when Winston Churchill and other British leaders started to think about how to rebuild their country after devastating losses. William Beveridge, a British aristocrat, is credited with developing the healthcare concept, based on his years of work championing social reforms. His idea: healthcare would be free to all and payment to doctors and hospitals would come through general taxation, not medical fees or insurance.[7] His plan was hugely popular at that critical moment in time, coming out of a shattering period of war and boosting the morale of an exhausted population. While his plan was opposed by many health groups, including doctors and insurers, the National Health Service was born and opened in 1948. (As a compromise, doctors were allowed to see patients on a private pay basis outside of the new government system, and insurers were still allowed to sell plans outside of the NHS, for people who wanted additional coverage.)

Since inception, the NHS care has been provided almost entirely for free, with few cost-sharing requirements. However, the NHS exerts a high degree of control over utilization of many of its health services in order to keep costs down: nobody gets to see a specialist until their primary care doctor approves it. The NHS also pays only for treatments it considers cost-effective. That said, everyone is assigned a primary care doctor, which helps with overall care coordination.

Britain has a zero percent uninsured rate. The country runs a very lean operation, spending only $4,246 per person annually on healthcare by tightly controlling how funds are spent. Even with this low spending, Britain has an infant mortality rate of 3.8 per thousand live births and a life expectancy of 81.2 years.

By contrast, as you'll see in the table in the next section, the US has an uninsured rate of 9 percent, an infant mortality rate of 5.9 per thousand live births, and a life expectancy of only 78.6 years.

CANADA

I felt that no boy should have to depend either for his leg or his life upon the ability of parents to raise enough money.

—TOMMY DOUGLAS, founder of Canadian single-payer system[8]

Canada has a federally sponsored *single-payer* system serviced by *private healthcare providers* that is called Medicare. Yes, it has the same name as the program in the US that insures the elderly, but Canada beat us to it, establishing the first portion of their Medicare program two decades before the US. Canada launched its universal healthcare system due to the passion of one man: Tommy Douglas, who served as the governor of Saskatchewan province in the 1940s. He was motivated by his own story, having been saved from a disabling injury by the chance benevolence of one doctor—his own family couldn't afford the surgery. The unfairness of that in relation to other children's situations troubled Douglas and led him to champion universal healthcare for his province.

Universal healthcare was established in Saskatchewan in 1947 (for hospital coverage only; physicians were added in 1962) and was so popular that the rest of Canada clamored for it. By 1961, Canada had implemented Medicare (for hospital coverage) for everyone in every province. By 1971, physician coverage was included.[9] Prescription drug coverage is one exception: outside of hospitals, it is only covered for certain populations, such as children, the elderly, and low-income people. Canadians can purchase additional coverage through the private sector (only for things the public system doesn't cover, such as drugs, dental, and vision)—two-thirds of Canadians have some form of private coverage.

Canada's Medicare program has centralized (federal) oversight and federal funds cover about half of spending. Similar to the role states play in the US Medicaid program, Canada's thirteen provinces and territories govern their own versions of Canada's Medicare program and cover the remainder of the public funding.[10] They also pay directly (or indirectly) for hospital care, negotiate physician rates, and administer prescription drug plans as well as long-term services and supports.

Canada has a zero percent uninsured rate. Canada manages to spend only $4,826 per capita annually on healthcare and has an infant mortality rate of 4.7 per thousand live births and life expectancy of 81.9 years.

GERMANY

The greatest burden for the working class is the uncertainty of life. They can never be certain they will have a job, or that they will have health and the ability to work. We cannot protect a man from all sickness and misfortune. But it is our obligation, as a society, to provide assistance when he encounters these difficulties. A rich society must care for the poor.

—OTTO VON BISMARCK, German chancellor and founder
of Germany's social health insurance system, 1884[11]

The German healthcare system was the world's first social health insurance system, which expanded over time to provide universal coverage. Established in 1883, it is a *public-private hybrid system*: it comprises a system of "sickness funds," which are *private nonprofit health insurance plans* that operate with strong government guidelines and purchase services from *private healthcare providers*. The insurance is not funded by general taxes—the premium-like contributions are a share of wages, paid equally by employers and employees, which are automatically deducted from paychecks (or included as part of unemployment benefits for those without jobs).[12] Germans have an individual mandate: they are required by law to be covered by the national system (i.e., one of 113 sickness funds) or they can opt out and buy their own private insurance (about 11 percent of people choose this).

The origins of the German universal healthcare system are interesting. The foundation was established by Otto von Bismarck, a fierce leader who ruled for over thirty years in the late 1800s and is credited with unifying Germany. He was known as the "Iron Chancellor," and historians have puzzled over what motivated him to establish such a humanitarian approach to health coverage. Some say it was practical politics, to win over a newly unifying population; others credit his Lutheran roots. Whatever the motivation, the system he established has endured and grown incrementally to provide universal coverage (full universal health coverage was achieved in 2009), and it has been copied by numerous other countries.

In the German system, people can buy private insurance to supplement their sickness fund (public) coverage for "extras," i.e., things that are above standard benefits, such as the opportunity to skip waiting lines, to have private rooms, or to obtain more services.[13] While sickness funds are always nonprofit, the private insurance funds can be for-profit. In the German model, surpluses get redistributed at the end of the year—insurers are there to pay bills, not make a profit.

Because Germans now get to choose their sickness fund, and the funds cannot turn people away or charge people more for their health conditions, they must compete on the elements of their products for which they are allowed flexibility in design, as well as a modest additional premium contribution. This has led to some innovative plans and has exerted downward pressure on pricing.[14]

The German system also features self-governing bodies representing doctors, dentists, hospitals, therapists, insurers, and the insured to represent their interests and ensure professional standards.[15] Despite the fact that the system is run by private entities, the government plays a critical role in setting the rules and guiding behavior.[16] It specifies which benefits are covered and requires doctors to join regional associations that negotiate contracts with sickness funds.[17] Germany controls provider and drug prices through global budgets and other mechanisms. And because of all of this, even with multiple payers, Germany has some single-payer attributes, in terms of fairness and simplicity—all patients are treated the same, there is a coordinated set of rules and forms, and provider fees are the same.[18]

Germany has a zero percent uninsured rate. Germany's health coverage is generous, has limited cost-sharing, and relatively high customer satisfaction.[19] The country spends $5,728 per person on healthcare, its infant mortality rate is 3.4 per thousand live births, and its life expectancy rate is 81.1 years.

Another interesting statistic from Germany is the low rate of emotional distress for women (defined as occasions when a woman experiences anxiety or great sadness that is difficult to cope with alone). It is only 7 percent, contrasted with 34 percent in the US. Germany's rate is actually the lowest among its peer nations.[20]

THE US IS OUTPERFORMED

Regardless of the approach they take to universal coverage, every developed country spends less than the US on healthcare yet outperforms the US on multiple measures of population health. It's worthwhile to look at how our results, and spending, compare to theirs. That way we can better understand our "return on investment."

In terms of investment, the US spends about twice as much per person on healthcare as other developed countries do, as shown in figure 9.1.

FIGURE 9.1 On average, other wealthy countries spend about half as much per person on health than the US spends.

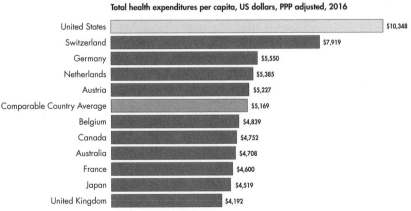

Total health expenditures per capita, US dollars, PPP adjusted, 2016

United States	$10,348
Switzerland	$7,919
Germany	$5,550
Netherlands	$5,385
Austria	$5,227
Comparable Country Average	$5,169
Belgium	$4,839
Canada	$4,752
Australia	$4,708
France	$4,600
Japan	$4,519
United Kingdom	$4,192

The US value was obtained from the 2016 National Health Expenditure data.

Source: Bradley Sawyer and Cynthia Cox, "How Does Health Spending in the U.S. Compare to Other Countries?," Peterson-Kaiser Health System Tracker, last updated December 7, 2018, https://www.healthsystemtracker.org.

Specifically, the US spends over $10,000 per person per year on health-care, which adds up to be about 18 percent of the total spending in our economy (also known as gross domestic product, or GDP). As we've seen, other developed countries such as Canada, Germany, and the United Kingdom spend $4,000 to $5,000 per person, or 9–11 percent of their GDP. This results in a wide gap with the US, and the gap has been growing.[21]

In terms of population health, table 9.1 summarizes the results for the three countries I described earlier, but they are similar for other developed nations (two of which I've included here—France and Denmark).

What's striking about this table is that it shows that Canada, Denmark, France, Germany, and the United Kingdom all

- Achieved universal healthcare coverage
- Spend far less on healthcare than the United States (which spends an astounding $10,209 per person annually)
- Attain better outcomes for their populations: their infant mortality rates are lower and their life expectancy rates are higher than those in the US. Their women's health measures are better as well, including lower maternal mortality rates (not shown here)

In sum, as T. R. Reid says, "No other industrialized democratic country allows people to die from treatable diseases because they can't afford the doctor's bill."[22] In fact, they spend less and get more.

These countries also reap other benefits, which are less commonly measured across countries. For example, no one goes bankrupt in other countries to pay for their healthcare. And with that financial health, comes much more peace of mind. Remember, Britain, Canada, and Germany each evolved their universal healthcare approaches differently. And each system has its own benefits and drawbacks. *But they all outperform the US.*[23]

H OW DID ALL of these other countries get to universal coverage? Most have made healthcare a right. When the European Union was created, the member countries adopted a Charter of Fundamental Rights, which says:

> Everyone has the right of access to preventive health care and the right to benefit from medical treatment under the conditions established by national law and practices. A high level of human health protection shall be ensured in the definition and implementation of all Union policies and activities.[24]

TABLE 9.1 A low return on investment: The US spends more on healthcare and less on social services than other wealthy nations and has worse population health outcomes.

Country	% Insured (A)[a]	% Gov't/ Social health insurance[b]	% Private health insurance[c]	GDP Per Capita[d]	Healthcare Spend per Capita ($)[e]	Healthcare Spend as a % of GDP[f]	% GDP spent on publicly funded social services and cash assistance[g]	Infant Mortality Rate (per 1,000 live births)[h]	Life Expectancy at Birth[i]
Canada	100.0	100.0	67.0	$48,300	$4,826	10.4%	17.3%	4.7	81.9
Denmark	100.0	100.0	32.5	$49,900	$5,183	10.2%	28.0%	3.1	80.9
France	99.9	99.9	...	$43,800	$4,902	11.5%	31.2%	3.7	82.4
Germany	100.0	89.3	33.9	$50,400	$5,728	11.3%	25.2%	3.4	81.1
UK	100.0	100.0	10.5	$44,100	$4,246	9.6%	20.6%	3.8	81.2
USA	90.9	36.3	63.0	$59,500	$10,209	17.1%	18.7%	5.9	78.6

Sources:

[a]"OECD Health Statistics," OECD iLibrary, https://www.oecd-ilibrary.org/social-issues-migration-health/data/oecd-health-statistics_health-data-en, doi: 10.1787/health-data-en.

[b]"OECD Health Statistics."

[c]"OECD Health Statistics."

[d]The World Factbook, Central Intelligence Agency, https://www.cia.gov/library/publications/the-world-factbook/rankorder/2004rank.html.

[e]"Health Spending," OECD Data, https://data.oecd.org/healthres/health-spending.htm.

[f]"Health Spending."

[g]"Compare Your Country," OECD, http://www.compareyourcountry.org/social-expenditure.

[h]"Infant Mortality Rates," OECD Data, https://data.oecd.org/healthstat/life-expectancy-at-birth.htm.

[i]"Life Expectancy at Birth," OECD Data, https://data.oecd.org/healthstat/life-expectancy-at-birth.htm.

(The charter is quite expansive—it also guarantees a right to paid parental leave and a clean environment, among other things.) Most European nations also adopted their own language making healthcare a right in their countries' constitution or laws.

They made that right into a reality by setting up or expanding their healthcare system to become a national system and opening it up to all legal residents. They took different approaches, based on their norms and values. Some, like Britain and Canada, make healthcare free and use government-contracted providers. Others, like Germany, collect payments from employers and employees on a sliding scale, and healthcare is provided through the private sector. Some, like Britain, were able to start from scratch. Others, like Canada and Germany, grew incrementally. Canada started with hospital coverage and added physician coverage later; Germany built on an existing system of "sickness" (insurance) funds and grew the coverage groups incrementally, until they got to universal coverage.

Americans tend to think about the healthcare systems in other developed countries as being at one extreme, achieving universal coverage only through 100 percent government-run single-payer programs (so-called socialized medicine). We tend to view the US system as being at the other extreme: an entirely free-market system with no government involvement at all. The reality is quite different. All of the countries I'm discussing—including the US—have some combination of public and private sector involvement—it's more a matter of degree. So, rather than being at one extreme or the other, we need to think of the different aspects of a healthcare system as being on a spectrum.

The degree of government involvement varies from country to country. Government involvement can include everything from government serving as the payer, to running the provider system, to simply regulating the payer and provider systems and negotiating prices. Britain and Canada have a high degree of government involvement in their healthcare systems. In contrast, the US has a mixed amount of government involvement: it is higher for government-sponsored public programs like Medicare and Medicaid, and much lower for private systems like employer-sponsored insurance (ESI). Germany's system falls somewhere in between the US public and private systems.

The number and type of payers also varies from country to country. Canada and Britain are at one end of the spectrum because they have a single payer (the government); at the other end of the spectrum is the American system of employer-sponsored insurance, which has multiple payers and little government involvement. In the middle of this spectrum are America's Medicaid and Medicare programs and Germany.

We need to throw out our conventional wisdom about what other countries are doing. It is not all "socialized (government-controlled) medicine" in the extreme sense. I would argue that for many countries, their universal healthcare system is government *supported*, or government *enabled*. Many countries have competitive elements, like the German sickness funds (private insurers), where consumers have plenty of choices. These countries have to make decisions about how much care to provide, but the decision about who receives it has already been made: it's everyone. To reiterate what one British health minister said, "We cover everybody, but we don't cover everything."

Another American criticism of so-called socialized medicine is that wait times for providers are longer than they are in the US. This is true in Canada (though it depends on the procedure) and sometimes Britain, but not in Germany; wait times in Germany are comparable or better than they are in the US.[25]

As for Americans' perception that countries with more government involvement in their healthcare systems have bloated bureaucracies, the reality is that their administrative costs as a percentage of healthcare spending are far less than those in the US. US health insurance companies spend at least 20 percent of their healthcare premiums on administration and nonmedical purposes (such as paperwork, reviewing claims, marketing, and profits); single-payer countries spend less than 5 percent. We Americans pay a price for our free-market system with its nonunified billing systems, spending on marketing, and in some cases, excessive profits.

UNIVERSAL HEALTHCARE IS NOT ENOUGH

After examining all of these approaches to universal healthcare and their results, I had a big "aha moment." As I dug deeper into this data, I discovered a discrepancy in our health outcomes, even for those in the US with excellent healthcare coverage. As I shared in chapter 7, it turns out that "the discrepancy in health between the US and its peer countries is apparent even among wealthy, well-educated, and white subgroups of the American public."[26] This went against what I had always thought, which was that health was tied to access to the healthcare system as well as socioeconomic status. This conventional wisdom is wrong—there's more than that driving our health.

I touched on many of these complexities in chapter 7, when I discussed the social determinants of health and rising inequality. Here's the key question: If other countries are getting better health outcomes for less money, does this mean they are doing a better job of spending their healthcare dollars? Or addressing the nonmedical factors (social determinants)? Or both?

PREVENTION

As the old saying goes, "An ounce of prevention is worth a pound of cure." Most other developed countries recognize this and emphasize preventive medical care rather than highly specialized care. Studies show that to fulfill the medical needs of a population, a country needs approximately 50–60 percent of its physicians to work in primary care.[27] In the United States, only 30 percent of physicians are practicing primary care and the numbers are declining: fewer than 20 percent of medical graduates are expected to enter primary care.[28] Compare this to France, where 65 percent of doctors practice general medicine,[29] or Germany, where approximately 46 percent are in primary care.[30] Although the US invests a relatively high dollar amount per person in prevention expenditures, the workforce and the structure of the healthcare system is underprepared to meet our primary care needs, especially as our population continues to age.[31]

Other countries also invest more in public health, which funds prevention activities for the whole population. One of government's jobs is to protect people, and investing in public health is a way to accomplish this. As T. R. Reid says, "Public health . . . can involve changing a nation's social and cultural norms on a massive scale."[32] Moreover, "Efforts to keep people healthy in the first place generally contribute more to the health of the entire population than the life-saving work of doctors treating individuals one by one."[33]

The US is paying a high price for underinvesting in these areas. Prevention saves lives. We don't pay enough attention to it in the US, and as a result, chronic diseases are a major cause of early deaths, and 40 percent of these early deaths are preventable.[34]

SOCIAL SERVICES

Comparisons with other countries point to another reason for the US' poor showing in health outcomes: other developed nations not only support universal healthcare and prevention, most also invest more in social services, many of which address the social determinants of health. Social services is a broad term here, encompassing direct service programs, such as education and job training, as well as income support programs, such as housing subsidies, unemployment insurance, and old-age assistance. These countries spend, on average, $2.29 on social services for every $1 spent on healthcare. By comparison, the US spends just $1.09 on social services for every $1 spent on healthcare. Figure 9.2 puts this into the context of total share of spending in the economy. For example, France and Denmark spend 31 percent and 28 percent of GDP, respectively, on publicly funded social programs; the US spends 19 percent.

As I showed in chapter 7, improving overall health means that we need to invest in addressing the social determinants of health, which means funding social services. The US underinvests in social services, and that hurts our health.

FIGURE 9.2 Health and Public Social Services Spending as a % of GDP by Country

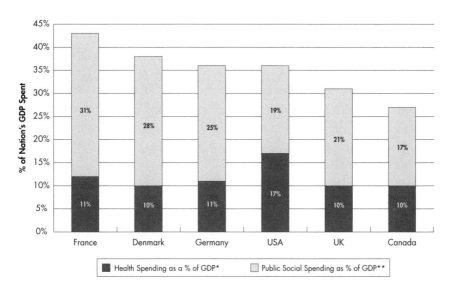

Source: "Social Spending," OECD, https://data.oecd.org/socialexp/social-spending.htm.

*Health spending measures the final consumption of healthcare goods and services (i.e., current health expenditure), including personal healthcare (curative care, rehabilitative care, long-term care, ancillary services, and medical goods) and collective services (prevention and public health services as well as health administration) but excluding spending on investments.

**Public social expenditure comprises cash benefits, direct in-kind provision of goods and services, and tax breaks with social purposes.

It seems counterintuitive that countries with universal healthcare also tend to pay a higher share of their income for social services. Shouldn't a government program that pays for everyone's healthcare cost so much that their public budgets would be strapped for cash, with barely any funds left for social services programs? Actually, an obligation to provide universal coverage means that social service programs make more financial sense. Let's step inside the shoes of Britain's National Health Service to see why.

The NHS is responsible for covering people for their entire lives. Everyone from newborns in the maternity ward to people in the workforce to retirees can be insured by the NHS until the day they die. The British government recognizes that investments in nonhealth programs, such as early childhood education or housing, made at age five will reduce health costs throughout many of the remaining seventy-five years of their expected life. Additional savings are realized in higher tax revenues and lower criminal justice costs, but one of the most compelling financial cases for these investments is in savings for the NHS.

Now consider the US. The US government is only on the hook for medical bills for a third of the population (those with Medicare or Medicaid coverage), resulting in a much-weakened financial incentive to make investments in the social determinants of health. And on the private side, insurers know that consumers hold their policies for only a few years. This severely weakens the financial case for private insurers to make these investments because before an investment pays off, their target population will have moved into another health plan and the investment ends up helping their competitor. The quarterly target mind-set employed by many private companies in this country certainly doesn't help.

WHAT OTHER COUNTRIES ARE DOING

Countries with universal healthcare are incented to take the longer view on investments that improve health. It's probably not a coincidence that many have made meaningful investments in education and social safety net programs that improve health outcomes. Here are just a few examples of the many approaches that other countries have taken.

Parental Leave: European countries guarantee at least fourteen weeks of *paid* maternity leave. The US only guarantees twelve weeks of *unpaid* leave, though California, New York, and, recently, Massachusetts provide a short-term disability benefit for maternity leave. The health benefits of paid leave

FIGURE 9.3 Every OECD Nation* besides the US Offers Paid Maternity Leave

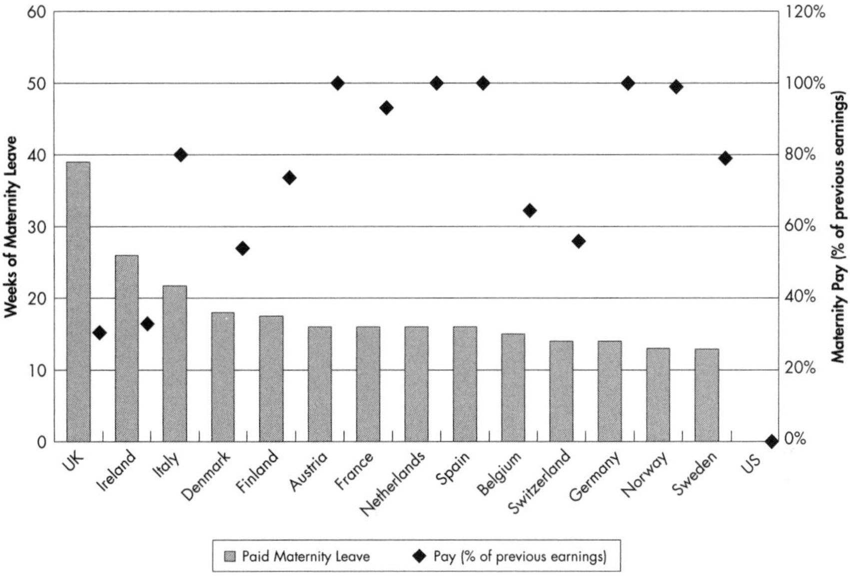

Sources:

"Which Countries in Europe Offer the Fairest Paid Leave and Unemployment Benefits?," Glassdoor.com, February 2016, https://www.glassdoor.com/research/app/uploads/sites/2/2016/02/GD_FairestPaidLeave_Final.pdf.

"PF2.1 Key characteristics of parental leave systems," OECD Family Database, last updated 2016, http://www.oecd.org/els/family/database.htm.

*Not all OECD nations shown in visual.

are significant. One study found that women who take paid maternity leave have a decrease in the odds of re-hospitalization of 53 percent for their children and 51 percent for them at twenty-one months postpartum.[35] More generous maternity leave following the birth of a first child has been shown to be associated with lower depression risk at old age.[36] (See figure 9.3.)

Subsidized Education: Most European countries provide at least two full years of free pre-primary education (before the age of five), and even make it a statutory right in most cases.[37] In the area of K–12 education, our peer nations spend less than the US does, but, just like with healthcare, they get better results.[38] One of the reasons for this is that although the average investment per student is high in the US, the quality of public K–12 education depends largely on the income and health of the community in which it is located—so the school system continues to perpetuate inequalities in society.[39] As noted in chapter 7, education impacts people's ability to navigate the healthcare system through increased literacy, including health literacy and numeracy. Additionally, education leads to attainment of economic resources, as well as access to social networks. Many other nations also invest more public dollars in higher education than the US, which funds higher education primarily with private funds. Most public colleges in the US are subsidized but are becoming increasingly expensive. In 1969, tuition in the University of California system was free. In 1975, it was $630 ($3,000 in 2019 US dollars). In 1995, it was $4,354 ($7,318 in 2019 US dollars). In 2009, it surpassed $10,000 (almost $12,000 in 2019 US dollars), and it's now $13,900.[40] Public universities in many other countries are more heavily subsidized, and they are often free. Sometimes the government will even provide a stipend for living expenses.

Unemployment Assistance: European countries have far more generous unemployment benefits than the US does, both in terms of dollar amount and duration. The dollar amount paid in the US depends on a person's former income, but the average paid is among the least generous in developed countries. The duration varies by state in the US—it's only fourteen weeks in some states. In Germany, unemployment benefits are available for at least one year; in France it's two years.[41]

GETTING FROM HERE TO THERE

If our ultimate goal is to improve health, then universal coverage is not enough. As I've said before, coverage is necessary, but not sufficient, for health. As we start developing solutions, it's important to look at the countries that are doing better than we are and learn from them. We can also look at successful programs in the US and expand them. The following are a few examples of both—these are best tackled comprehensively, at the national level, but state-level action can help too.

Earned Income Tax Credit: One of the most successful antipoverty initiatives the US has ever enacted, and one of the easiest tools to tap, is the earned income tax credit, which provides some extra income to low-wage workers at the end of every year. It could be expanded to lower-middle-income workers both nationally and at the state level. It's a program with bipartisan support, and it now provides more benefits than food stamps.

Food Stamps: Now called the Supplemental Nutrition Assistance Program (SNAP), this program provides subsidies to low-income people to buy food. The program has had an enormous impact on health. SNAP benefits cost the government approximately $1,548 per recipient per year. Participation in the program is associated with a $1,409 decrease in average annual healthcare costs.[42] Essentially, the program pays for itself in reduced healthcare expenditures. When you factor in the money from these benefits that circulates through the economy due to the spending of low-income SNAP beneficiaries, the program has a great return on investment.

Education: Our education system is the "drawbridge to the American dream," and it is not performing well for low-income students. In addition, college has become less accessible. This means our educational outcomes are increasingly influenced by income rather than by intelligence and hard work, exacerbating inequality and hurting our health. Solving this is beyond the scope of this book, but there are many innovative programs that can be expanded. One of my favorite emerging ideas is to support a new GI-like bill that would link free college opportunities to national service.

To sum up, there are three main things that other countries are doing differently that give them better health outcomes than those of the US. The first is that they all have universal healthcare. The second is that they've made commitments to support prevention, including preventive medicine and public health. And finally, they tend to invest more in social services.

There is plenty to learn in each of these areas, but in keeping with this book's focus on universal coverage, I'll turn to what we can learn from other countries' approaches to the design and implementation of a universal coverage system. Here are the key takeaways: First, the countries have made healthcare a right. Second, they have developed approaches to universal coverage that fit their values and norms (for them, that includes relying on either government or nonprofits to deliver a lot of their coverage and care). Third, the universal coverage is government enabled, with the government's role in financing and providing health services ranging from moderately significant to very significant. Fourth, many got there incrementally. These key elements can be used as a high-level framework for a universal coverage solution in the US, which I'll return to in the next chapters.

That said, as much as these other countries have achieved, it's important to recognize that their approaches aren't perfect. Many of these countries view themselves as being in a constant state of "health reform," which means they are continually refining their approach. They have to—they experience the push and pull of politics in ways similar to those that Americans do. And they are accountable for consumer satisfaction.

For example, in Britain, the satisfaction with the NHS has been waning in recent years due to insufficient funding. The strict regulation of services has always been a sticking point for those who want more freedom in seeking services and providers.[43] And in Canada, in spite of the good health outcomes, 55 percent of Canadians believe their health system needs fundamental change or rebuilding.[44] The main source of patient dissatisfaction is provider wait times, especially for people living in cities, people needing primary care in shortage areas, and those seeking specialty services. Germans, on the other hand, are happier with their healthcare system when compared to most other countries: only 37 percent believe it needs fundamental change or rebuilding.[45]

Compared to the US, however, citizens of these countries wouldn't trade their healthcare system for ours. In no other developed nation are people dying or going bankrupt because they don't have adequate insurance coverage. These countries have made the commitment to cover everyone, and that's nonnegotiable.

In terms of specifics, the German model in particular has many elements we could adopt in the US. In fact, more countries have adopted Germany's (Bismarck) model than England's single-payer model (including France, the Netherlands, Belgium, Switzerland, and Japan). They all use a system of private insurers and private providers, with their governments regulating coverage and pricing to varying degrees.

Unfortunately, Americans are often reluctant to learn from other countries. I've been fortunate to travel in and be educated about what other countries are doing, but most Americans don't have this opportunity. Without the true knowledge of what others are doing, we can get stuck in our own conventional wisdom. And, unfortunately, overzealous patriotism can also get in the way so that we believe "we are the best," no matter what.

One of the easiest ways to dismiss the opportunity to learn from other countries is to assume that "those people" are too different from us, too foreign. Or that we are too different because our country is larger and has a more diverse population than other countries. Certainly, America's extremes in inequality (racially, economically) make reaching solutions more challenging. But there's more to it than that.

Extensive research shows that key core values for many countries with universal healthcare are not that different from those of the US. For example, many of these countries embrace competition and free-market principles; they also value freedom. In addition, they have increasingly diverse populations. At the same time, they value solidarity and believe that government should help those in need. The systems they have designed reflect those values and are accommodating the diversity. It makes sense to learn from them.

Interestingly, for as little as we may be willing to learn from other countries, several of the patches on our US coverage quilt already reflect a variety of "foreign" models: our Medicare system is similar to Canada's in that government finances it, sets the prices, and provides uniform coverage, and it is privately run; we cover our military and Native Americans with a government-provided system that resembles England's; and our ACA exchanges and Medicare Advantage systems offer competing private insurance plans subject to government guidelines, which is similar to Germany's approach.

THE UNITED STATES LIKES to think of itself as an "exceptional" country. But American exceptionalism has gone in the wrong direction for healthcare coverage. Our healthcare costs are too high, and our access is too low. All of the other industrialized nations provide universal healthcare. We are exceptional because we do *not* do this.

A universal healthcare system combined with strong social supports has improved the quality of life and the value of healthcare spending in other countries. There are many ways that universal healthcare could look in the US. To design the system, we must answer a lot of questions about how to fund and operationalize it, plus find a way to sync it with our values. Who will get healthcare? What are the limitations on the services we provide? What do we spend our limited resources on? These are important questions. But we don't have to have all of these answers in order to take the next steps.

We should aspire to be a global leader in health outcomes. We can get there if we get smarter about these issues and then address them. We need universal coverage *and* more investment in social services. As Bradley and

Taylor say, "Changing the dialogue around health to be holistic and inclusive of nonmedical contributions is paramount to resolving the spend more, get less phenomenon in American health care."[46]

If we do that, then we will get the type of value for our healthcare dollar that people get in comparable industrialized nations. That day won't come, however, without our involvement and activism. We can play a critical role in advocating for changes to our system, because what is abundantly clear is that the system we have right now isn't working. Let's turn next to some potential solutions. There's urgency to do so—people are dying while we wait.

CHAPTER 10

EXPANDING HEALTHCARE ACCESS AND AFFORDABILITY

Women belong in all the places decisions are being made.

—JUSTICE RUTH BADER GINSBURG[1]

I CAN STILL SEE THE SIGNS and hear the chants from the Women's Marches: "Healthcare is a human right!" And it's not just the marchers saying this: 92 percent of Americans believe that healthcare is a right.[2] Getting 92 percent of Americans to agree on anything is an incredible feat—only 74 percent of Americans agree that the Earth revolves around the sun instead of vice versa.[3] There is a shared belief in this country that everyone deserves healthcare regardless of income or background. But what does this mean, exactly? Evolving this concept from a stump speech refrain into guaranteeing healthcare coverage for all has proven to be difficult politically, especially because of the enormous cost of providing healthcare in this country.

Even the way that healthcare coverage is discussed has become politically charged, so much so that a term such as *single-payer* suggests bias. I'll use *universal coverage* as a neutral term to describe access to affordable healthcare for all. This is why we see such consensus around the idea of healthcare as a right; *access* pulls on political heartstrings on both sides of the political aisle because it is part of our imagined principles of healthcare in the United States. And for good reason. The consequences of low coverage rates are severe—Americans face too many avoidable deaths and bankruptcies. As we've seen, people who are uninsured are at a much higher risk of death.[4] And, as T. R. Reid puts it, many Americans are just "one diagnosis away from financial ruin."[5]

So why is expanding access so difficult? Part of the reason is that, as I explained in chapter 8, healthcare reforms have to make their way through a politically polarized environment and, unfortunately, both political parties tend to downplay the downsides of their ideas. Republicans tend to downplay the consequences of low levels of coverage and overstate the ability of the free market to address them. Democrats tend to downplay the cost of providing coverage through government-sponsored programs. Solving the problems of healthcare coverage in this country requires a nuanced approach and careful consideration of the societal and budgetary ramifications of the solution.

CAN OUR FREE-MARKET SYSTEM GET US THERE?

Although support for government-sponsored healthcare has grown substantially in the United States,[6] many still believe that the invisible hand of the free market will produce the best outcome. This simply isn't true, if universal coverage is our goal. The first problem with this idea is that a pure market allows those with money to purchase things and leaves out the rest. For people with an illness or a preexisting condition, not being able to purchase health insurance can have severe, potentially life-threatening consequences compared to not being able to buy a commodity like a car.

The second problem (as I discussed in chapter 2) is that healthcare functions differently from a traditional market—many economists even use the term "market failure" to describe certain aspects of the healthcare system. Among them is the famous economist Kenneth Arrow, who made this diagnosis in the 1950s. Remember, the risk pool incentives are greatly skewed between insurers and consumers, which throws off the supply and demand equation. And because insurance shields consumers from prices, buyers tend to overconsume, and sellers are able to charge more. In addition, the power of market share lends advantage to larger insurers.

These facts about the health insurance market make a compelling case for government intervention, since only the government can make rules to remedy these market failures and ensure high levels of coverage via direct coverage programs, subsidization, and/or coverage mandates. Just as significantly, government is already a purchaser for a large portion of the US healthcare market, via Medicare and Medicaid.

These important roles for government lead to this question: what should government intervention in the healthcare industry look like if our goal is universal coverage? As I showed in chapter 9, most other developed nations have higher degrees of government involvement in their healthcare system than the United States. Approaches vary: some countries have the highest level of government involvement, which is single-payer healthcare, and some countries have a hybrid government-private sector model. Let's look at the models that are being proposed in the US, and where they fit in the spectrum of government involvement.

SINGLE-PAYER COVERAGE

In conversations about "universal coverage," people often start talking about "single-payer" healthcare, and they frequently use the terms interchangeably. I want to make it clear that "single-payer" does not mean "universal coverage." Also, a single-payer system is not required to get to universal coverage. Let's take a deeper dive into what single-payer really means.

The definition of single-payer is a healthcare system in which one entity—a single payer—collects all healthcare fees and pays for all healthcare costs. The single-payer entity is usually the government and the fees are usually some form of taxes. In the US, (traditional) Medicare is a single-payer system.[7]

Support for a single-payer system in the United States has been growing in recent years: currently, 51 percent of Americans support a government-run single-payer plan.[8] Democratic candidates are increasingly talking about the issue in their "Medicare for All" proposals. That said, there appears to be a great deal of confusion on the issue. And support declines when people are told their taxes will rise to pay for it.[9]

The single-payer healthcare systems of other industrialized nations have strong track records in terms of cost and health outcomes, and there are certain advantages to such a system. For instance, the biggest way that single-payer systems can keep costs down for consumers is that they can set or negotiate lower prices from healthcare providers. A single-payer by definition holds a monopoly (100 percent market share), so the payer can set or negotiate much lower rates with providers.

Single-payer systems can also keep costs down by being more operationally efficient. It's ironic, since most people in the US don't think of government as being efficient. But having just one payer means there's only one entity that medical claims are sent to, one universal system for processing them, and one set of rules about what is covered. It's much simpler than our current system, where providers must juggle multiple contracts, billings, and incentives tied to each contract, and consumers must undergo eligibility determination processes for public programs. A single payer would also use a single, integrated operational and information technology system instead of each insurer developing its own. Britain's national health system runs this way, and its administrative expenses are about one-fifth of the US healthcare system's.[10]

In addition, in a single-payer system, certain insurance company roles like sales and account management would no longer be necessary and profit would no longer be made from insurance—all of the financing would instead be paying for healthcare and the leaner administrative costs of running the system. So while there would still be administrative costs, they would be far lower than they are in our private insurance system today—estimates are around 6 percent, which is much closer to Medicare's 3 percent level.[11]

Naturally, there are certain disadvantages to single-payer systems. For instance, most healthcare providers will dislike a single-payer system if their payment rates are lower. Their potentially lower rates would be somewhat mitigated by the fact that providers would have access to a larger patient pool and would be stuck with fewer unpaid bills. Nonetheless, healthcare providers in the US have typically balked at single-payer proposals.

Another big group that could lose in a single-payer system would be insurers, depending on the single-payer model adopted. If the model is like traditional Medicare, then insurers might subcontract with the government to be the "back office" of the single-payer system, administering payments and managing data, but their role and income would be significantly reduced from what they are today. If the model is like the Medicare Advantage portion of Medicare, then private insurers could play their more traditional role of competing for enrollees, but the market would be highly regulated, with defined, and most likely lower, payment rates.[12]

Consumers might also lose, if they are worried that "government-controlled healthcare" will lead to harsh rationing, such as denied treatments, or long wait times to see doctors. These are not necessarily by-products of a single-payer system but can be mistaken for such. (Important note: rationing already takes place in a free-market system—it just happens by price, i.e., limiting care for those unable to pay.)

The specter of these potential problems for healthcare providers, insurers, and consumers has prevented the US from adopting a single-payer healthcare system. The closest we have come was nearly a century ago. Franklin Roosevelt tried to include such a system as a provision of the Social Security Act of 1935 but later removed it out of fear that interest-group opposition, primarily from physicians, would derail the whole bill.[13] Fourteen years later, President Truman sent a message to Congress to push for a single-payer system, but neither of the two resulting bills, which were again subject to strong interest-group opposition led by physicians in the American Medical Association, managed to pass or even came to votes in either the House or Senate.[14]

These two opportunities, if even partially realized, could have put the United States on a course to universal coverage, but we missed the chance. In the subsequent decades, private insurance became more established across the market, while the costs of medical care rose faster than incomes. Now moving to single-payer would require an overhaul of this $3.65 trillion industry, including addressing the immense variation in payments made to providers by different payers. And yet, the appetite for single-payer is strong among a certain segment and is fueling a growing popular movement for a universal coverage solution in the US. Single-payer activists are gaining support by imagining a coverage solution that is as widely accepted and valued as Social Security and Medicare.

H OW WOULD WE GET TO SINGLE-PAYER TODAY? Many experts believe that the most politically and operationally feasible way to achieve any form of universal coverage would be to expand Medicare or Medicaid. Of the several single-payer bills that have been introduced in recent years, Vermont senator and presidential candidate Bernie Sanders's Medicare for All has gotten the most attention. He introduced it in 2017 (similar to bills he filed in prior sessions) and reintroduced it in 2019 as part of his presidential campaign. The bill represents one approach to single-payer, and it is a useful case to study because several credible sources have analyzed the bill and developed cost projections. His bill starts with the foundation of the current Medicare program, since Medicare already covers forty-five million people and wouldn't need to be built from scratch—though Sanders's proposal differs in many substantial ways from the current structure of Medicare. It is exceptionally generous, with no out-of-pocket expenses and with added benefits (dental, vision, and hearing coverage). It also expands support for long-term care services. These proposed benefits are far more generous than the system it was meant to emulate, Canada's Medicare program. At the same time, it proposes paying healthcare providers at Medicare's current-law rates, which can average anywhere from 25 percent to 40 percent less than they currently receive from commercial payers.[15] Even with these lower rates, Medicare for All's total estimated cost averages at least $4 trillion per year over a ten-year period. Most experts project it will require between $2.4 trillion and $2.8 trillion in new revenues each year.[16]

To put these astronomical numbers in perspective:

- In 2018 the federal government collected a total of $3.3 trillion in revenue.[17]
- Medicare, which is already considered to be a huge federal program, costs "only" $705 billion per year.[18]
- The total value of all employer-sponsored insurance payments (from employers and employees) is over $1 trillion per year.[19] A single-payer system would require shifting these expenses to the government and raising revenues to cover them.
- The US' GDP is currently $19.5 trillion and grows 1.5–3 percent per year.

This last factoid is important to note. It means that, under Sanders's plan, healthcare would remain at its current expenditure rate of 18 percent of the GDP if averaged over the next ten years. That means that the US wouldn't benefit from the decreased costs experienced by other single-payer countries, who spend only about 10 percent of their GDP on healthcare.

Why can't the US achieve this lower spending level that other countries do when using a universal coverage system? There are many reasons, the biggest one being that Americans pay significantly higher prices for healthcare services.[20] The bottom line is that we can't transition to a Medicare for All system by simply snapping our fingers and cutting our healthcare costs to the level that other single-payer systems spend. In theory, a single-payer system could exert downward pressure on healthcare costs in the United States little by little. Over time, the health-spending-as-a-percent-of-GDP would then fall to the levels of other countries. But this could take decades, since our healthcare system is so large and entrenched in the way it does business. Making these changes would certainly disrupt providers and the delivery of care to patients. And paying for the system during this period of adjustment would require an enormous amount of new revenue.

Many states, including California, Colorado, Iowa, Ohio, New York, and Vermont have introduced single-payer bills.[21] None of these bills have passed except for Vermont's. Most of these bills were introduced with little expectation of passage. This may be changing. Public support of single-payer health plans is on the rise, and is higher among younger generations.[22] The increasing awareness of the advantages of such a system, combined with an escalating sense of urgency engendered by the rapidly rising price of health insurance, has led to an increase in legislation that proposes single-payer systems in various forms.

That said, Vermont's attempt to implement single-payer is a cautionary tale. Vermont forayed into state single-payer in 2010 with a system called Green Mountain Care. However, after a series of setbacks and a costly political battle, Green Mountain Care was abandoned.[23] Among the reasons for Bernie Sanders's own state giving up on its single-payer program was its high costs—there was an anticipated increase in the state budget of 45 percent— and insufficient public support.

In sum, implementing a single-payer system in the US would be a tremendous challenge. The trillions of dollars in government costs are daunting, even if private healthcare spending by households and employers was reduced dramatically. Which brings up another issue: requiring half of the population to leave an employer-sponsored insurance program would likely be a nonstarter for millions, and nearly half of Americans are unaware that's what would be required.[24] In addition, negative perceptions (and misperceptions) of government-run programs make universal expansion politically difficult. Add to this the entrenched interests of the healthcare industry, and it becomes clear that implementing single-payer systems is a politically costly fight to take on. As Yale political scientist Jacob Hacker says, "It would be hard to design a less welcoming context for single-payer. Enacting a universal program meant taking on a lobbying juggernaut to impose taxes on people generally suspicious of government, most of whom were insulated from the true costs of their care."[25] Not to mention the fact that every US president who has attempted to do so has seen a decline in support.

So, if it's not single-payer, how do we get to universal coverage?

A public-private hybrid program, meaning a mix of government and private sector elements, would be more politically feasible than single-payer. A public-private hybrid program may also be able to draw from some benefits of a single-payer system without requiring a huge transition—taking some of the best of both worlds. Let's explore what it might look like.

A PUBLIC-PRIVATE HYBRID SOLUTION

As I discussed in chapter 9, health coverage system approaches are on a couple of spectrums, reflecting the degree of government involvement and the number of payers. At one end is a universal, government-run single-payer program; at the other end is a free market, completely private insurance system. Each one has its drawbacks. Rather than seeing this as an "either/ or" issue, we need to think about hybrid possibilities in the middle. And in fact, America already falls in the middle of these spectrums with some of its coverage programs.

The Medicaid and Medicare programs are actually hybrids themselves, containing some government involvement and some private sector elements. The Medicaid, CHIP, and Medicare Advantage programs all contract with private insurers to provide coverage. (Medicare Advantage, also known as Medicare Part C, allows consumers to select a private insurance plan. This market-based approach was greatly expanded by a 2003 law championed by President George W. Bush.) Finally, the health insurance exchanges set up by the Affordable Care Act, including Healthcare.gov, are another example of this hybrid approach in the US, offering multiple private insurer options with government supports and guardrails.

Since the hybrid approach to coverage is already established in much of our healthcare system, it could form the basis for expanded coverage. We could expand this blended system in which private enterprise has a role and the government establishes the guardrails needed to avoid market failure and ensure high coverage levels.

I'll explore four emerging examples of this hybrid approach that are worth considering: a public option program (based on Medicare), a whole new public program, and two proposals that allow people to buy into existing programs (Medicare and Medicaid).

EXAMPLE #1: A MEDICARE-BASED PUBLIC OPTION

Yale professor Jacob Hacker developed an idea of how to build upon the current Medicare program by creating a new component that would serve as a *public option*, called *Medicare Part E* (*E* is for "everyone"). (A public option means that the general public would be allowed to purchase a government-run health plan, like Medicare or Medicaid, even if they don't belong to the current groups of eligible people—elderly, disabled, or low income.) Medicare Part E as proposed would cover hospitals and care facilities, doctors, and pharmacy expenses—services currently covered by Medicare Parts A, B, and D (for more information on Medicare, see the glossary). Here's where Medicare Part E differs from single-payer: the Medicare Part E plan would compete with private insurance. In Hacker's original conception, people would be automatically enrolled in Part E and could switch to an alternative private plan, as long as it met minimum standards, and employers would be required to provide either compliant coverage or contribute to Medicare to fund it.[26] (In the bills that have been filed using Hacker's ideas, the actual provisions have varied.)

A public option such as Hacker's model wouldn't be able to exert the same amount of downward price pressures that a single-payer system could apply. However, it would still have an effect. By allowing Medicare to compete with private insurance, the program's comparatively lower prices would likely push prices down for everyone. Our healthcare industry couldn't handle a sudden 40 percent drop in reimbursement, anyway (as Medicare for All calls for). This option would instead slowly constrain the growth of healthcare costs and result in less shock to the delivery system.

Several pieces of federal legislation have been introduced for various versions of this option. One example is the Choose Medicare Act, filed by Democratic senators Jeff Merkley (Oregon) and Chris Murphy (Connecticut), which opens up Medicare as a public option plan to all Americans, including employers. It builds on the ACA framework: it would be sold on the ACA exchanges, use the ACA subsidy structures, and preserve the ACA's protections for preexisting conditions. The bill would provide more generous tax credits and eligibility thresholds than those currently in the ACA. It addresses cost control by allowing Medicare to negotiate prices for prescription drugs.

The upshot: A Medicare-based public option is a possible path to universal coverage.

EXAMPLE #2: A WHOLE NEW PUBLIC PROGRAM,
WITH PRIVATE MARKET COMPONENTS

There are also proposals to create a whole new public program with private market components: one is called Medicare for America. (The name is a bit confusing, since it uses "Medicare," but it actually sets up a new program.) Sponsored by Democratic representatives Rosa DeLauro (Connecticut) and Jan Schakowsky (Illinois), the program has a lot of the elements of Medicare Part E described above, including automatically enrolling all US citizens, with no eligibility determination process. It allows people to keep their employer-sponsored insurance, but gives them the option to purchase a Medicare for America plan, and gives their employers that option as well. Private insurance plans can compete, similar to the Medicare Advantage program. Enrollees must pay some of the premium costs, but deductibles would be capped, and cost-sharing would be based on income at levels that are more generous than those of the ACA. It addresses cost control by allowing Medicare for America to negotiate prices for prescription drugs. In addition, it would enroll people who are currently eligible for Medicaid, CHIP, and Medicare, and it would allow some generous benefits, such as long-term care services. Finally, the fact that it automatically enrolls newborns means that over a long period of time it would likely replace the current employer-sponsored insurance system.

Another idea for a stand-alone public program with private market components is the Healthy America program developed by several Urban Institute fellows.[27] This option builds broadly on the ACA framework too. It would offer new, affordable insurance options for those who need them by creating a new government-enabled program with a widely accessible public option, along with competing private insurance options, while still allowing people to keep their employer-sponsored insurance. It would provide more generous subsidies than the ACA does, and would enroll people under age sixty-five who are currently eligible for Medicaid. It would control costs by capping provider payment rates and requiring drug rebates from manufacturers, to lower drug prices.

The upshot: A new public program, with private market components, is another possible path to univeral coverage.

EXAMPLE #3: "MIDLIFE MEDICARE"

A less ambitious proposal for Medicare expansion has been named by its proponent, Princeton professor Paul Starr, "Midlife Medicare."[28] This would allow people over the age of fifty to purchase Medicare. While not a universal coverage proposal, it would grow the coverage patch of Medicare. Presumably those ages fifty to sixty-five would like this extra option. Starr suggests that seniors and the American Association of Retired Persons (AARP), a powerful lobbying organization representing people age fifty and over, would be more likely to accept Midlife Medicare because those fifty and up have already paid into the Medicare program, and because the AARP represents this constituency.

The program could also lower prices for the individual market, because it would remove the older and sicker population from its risk pools. However, it could risk alienating millennials, who would be asked to apply their tax dollars toward yet another program for which they don't enjoy the full benefits. (Millennials will be eligible for Medicare later in life, but if the program's solvency issues aren't resolved, they will ultimately receive much less than they paid into the program in their younger years.)

Senator Debbie Stabenow of Michigan has filed a "Medicare at 50" bill that essentially embraces a similar idea.[29]

The upshot: Because "Midlife Medicare" is targeted only to one age bracket, it would need to be combined with other solutions to get to universal coverage.

EXAMPLE #4: "MEDICAID FOR MORE"

The country would have a head start, as with the Medicare-based examples, if it were to use the Medicaid program as the foundation for universal coverage. Medicaid is the largest insurer in the US—it already covers over sixty million people. States could expand their Medicaid programs by establishing a buy-in option. This would allow expansion to happen incrementally, state-by-state, rather than requiring a revamp of the entire US healthcare coverage system at once. Medicaid can be expanded through state legislation, and states are often more flexible and willing to experiment. State-specific designs could be tailored to each state's needs, so the transition might incur less political controversy from that standpoint.

Medicaid has lots of experience expanding coverage to new populations: it has gradually expanded over the past three decades to cover more and more people, as with the ACA's Medicaid expansion and the forty states that now allow people with disabilities to buy in to the program.[30] The mixed federal-state funding mechanism has worked well for the program to date, providing flexibility with economic changes, and its low cost would make it highly competitive.

In 2017, Nevada passed a Medicaid buy-in law that would have allowed residents to buy a Medicaid plan on the state's exchange (such a system would only be possible in the states that run their own marketplace exchanges).[31] The bill didn't make it past the Republican governor's desk, but others may try again.[32] At the federal level, Democratic senator Brian Schatz (Hawaii) proposed a Medicaid buy-in bill in late 2017 and reintroduced it in early 2019.[33] Other states will be watching these events closely, pondering whether they might be able to pull off a Medicaid buy-in program.

The drawbacks to attempting universal coverage on a state-by-state basis through Medicaid is that the program wouldn't be able to leverage a single centralized structure to achieve cost and operational efficiencies. In addition, doctors and hospitals would balk at being paid Medicaid's very low rates for more of their patients—this would certainly generate political controversy. Moreover, many states would likely choose not to opt into the program, so we wouldn't get to true universal coverage without mandating some level of benefits (a near impossibility, given that the US Supreme Court ruled in 2012 that the federal government cannot mandate state participation in major Medicaid changes). Finally, the Medicaid program is more vulnerable to funding cuts than the Medicare program is, typically from "block granting" proposals that would cap federal funding to states.

The upshot: Medicaid for More would leave us with a continued patchwork quilt and many bare spots.

A RECOMMENDED SOLUTION

In reviewing these examples, I'm drawn to many of the good ideas in the Medicare for America and Healthy America proposals, which bring together some of the best elements of what works in Medicare and the ACA. Both proposals would allow people to keep their employer-sponsored insurance and both maintain a role for private insurers while providing a robust public coverage alternative through a new public-private hybrid program, whether it's called Medicare or something else. I like this concept, not only because it is less disruptive to people who want to keep coverage through their employer and because it gives people choices, but also because employer-sponsored insurance provides an important alternative to government coverage and can challenge government to innovate in its approach (for example, by embracing value-based insurance design and centers of excellence). Both programs also include some form of auto-enrollment, which helps ensure everyone gets covered.

To get to a universal healthcare solution, it's best to start with what's working elsewhere (such as in another state or another country) and borrow those ideas, just as the ACA's designers did with the Massachusetts health reform model. In chapter 9 we saw that other countries have achieved universal healthcare using different approaches. We found those difference don't matter on one level, given that each of these countries has achieved much better population health results than those of the US. That said, the differences are worth examining. And the approach does matter. To have ongoing political support, a program has to be in sync with that country's norms and values.

Given America's norms and values, the US needs a universal healthcare solution that blends both the public and private sector roles, incorporating the best of each. Other nations have done this. Their governments ensure baseline coverage (think fleece blanket) for everyone, and yet people can (and do) choose to purchase private insurance *in addition to* the coverage provided by the government.

We can begin by finding a way to combine the best elements of our current public and private sector healthcare coverage systems. We can choose an existing government program to serve as the baseline of coverage and the fallback plan. We can then incorporate the key elements that support our values, which will be discussed more fully in the next chapter. We also need to include operational tools, such as auto-enrollment, so we have a default plan that provides a true safety net for families and individuals, so they don't have to get tied up in unnecessary administrative complexity. This is essential when you consider that over a quarter of uninsured people are eligible for the current healthcare programs Medicaid and CHIP. In addition, we should include certain primary and preventive care services in baseline coverage, *before* any deductible has to be met. We also have to recognize that the universal health solution cannot cover everything. For example, unproven drugs and procedures can be extremely costly and may need to be accessed through supplemental insurance.

The most feasible path for coverage expansion in this country is not to toss out our threadbare quilt and replace it with a new one, as Medicare for All would do, but rather to grow and reinforce the pieces we currently have. The "growing the pieces" method could be a longer, less direct path to attaining affordable universal coverage, and will be less effective at containing costs. But it's more feasible. In addition, we need to focus on healthcare affordability for all, not just increasing coverage—the audience for mobilizing the universal healthcare solution would be much bigger, since this is such a huge "kitchen table" issue. In so doing, we should think about ways to provide a fleece blanket layer to everyone, meaning a seamless coverage program that provides comfort and can stretch. It would guarantee minimum coverage (including primary care and prevention services) and a safety net for all.

No matter what, all of these options will have to be reviewed in light of ways of financing them, which I will address in chapter 11.

IN THE MEANTIME, STRENGTHEN THE ACA

We can't forget about the Affordable Care Act while we are exploring universal coverage options. The ACA has covered millions of people and protected millions more who have preexisting conditions. It provides a key link between the public and private systems of health coverage in the US. It can serve as an important building block on the path to universal healthcare because it enables many key principles that Americans hold dear, such as consumer choice. It supports the private insurance market, while also regulating it for fairness, access, and affordability. So, as part of our efforts to enact universal coverage, we should strengthen and expand the ACA to cover more people and reduce the level of underinsurance by making insurance in the individual market more affordable.

To do this, we must address the ACA's original shortcomings and reverse the actions that have been taken to undermine it. As discussed in chapter 5, the ACA had three major shortcomings: it was not affordable enough, it did not control costs enough, and it was not well understood. Combined, these shortcomings in design and implementation had the effect of not achieving universal coverage. To address the shortcomings and strengthen the ACA, we should lobby for the following improvements to the current law, at the state and federal levels: increase subsidies to make insurance affordable for more people, restore the individual mandate, and expand outreach. (For more info on these ideas, and some wonky ways to get there, see my website, https://rosemarieday.com.)

Massachusetts senator and presidential candidate Elizabeth Warren filed a bill in early 2018 to strengthen the ACA by doing most of these things. Her bill would help more people who don't have employer-sponsored insurance buy coverage on the ACA marketplaces. In addition to increasing premium subsidies and capping out-of-pocket costs, it would set stronger limits on insurer profits and require insurers to spend a larger share of the premium dollar on healthcare.[34] In early 2019, the House of Representatives, under Speaker Nancy Pelosi, proposed a package of fixes to the ACA that included most of these things as well. And in 2019, California passed a law combining the ACA's original carrot-and-stick approaches; it significantly increased subsidies for people buying health insurance through the state exchange, Covered California, and established an individual mandate to buy health insurance.

Throughout these efforts, we need to continue to spread the word about the ACA's benefits. When the ACA passed, many Americans stood to gain from its provisions, even though they may not have understood that initially. Remarkably, the threat of ACA repeal has been one of the biggest sources of education about the ACA for the general public: it certainly helped people realize what protections for preexisting conditions mean, in a way that they didn't before. This has led to some interesting side effects, including the fact that ACA opponents are now saying they support the newly popular protections for people with preexisting conditions (even if they don't yet appear to have a credible plan to achieve this outside of the ACA).

These measures to strengthen the ACA stand in sharp contrast to Republicans' approach to making insurance more affordable. Most of their proposals find ways around the ACA's protections and go back to the days of selling cheap insurance to healthy people. But even so, one of the ACA's shortcomings was that it did not do enough to control costs. We need to tackle this. Polls indicate that reducing healthcare costs is a concern for everyone, regardless of party affiliation. So we need to find some bipartisan common ground here. Reducing healthcare costs won't be enough of a galvanizing issue on its own, but it could be combined with other universal coverage solution pieces that generate enthusiasm. (I address this further in chapter 11.)

Strengthening the ACA requires addressing all three legs of the stool described in chapter 5, keeping the balance of shared responsibility among insurers, government, and individuals. Each of these ACA enhancements would create another incremental solution which would strengthen pieces of the patchwork quilt of coverage and address major pain points as expressed by Americans when asked about the insecurity of their health insurance.

Whether the ACA on its own can achieve truly universal coverage is a good question. Massachusetts, which led the way with the model for the ACA, has achieved "near-universal" coverage, with an uninsured rate that is currently 3 percent. The state's exchange subsidies are more generous than the ACA's, and so is its Medicaid program. Increasing subsidies for all ACA exchanges would certainly bring in millions more people to coverage. And simply expanding Medicaid in the states that haven't yet done so could cover up to 2.5 million of the 28 million remaining uninsured. There would still be gaps, however—without additional changes, the expanded programs won't reach everyone who's eligible. That's because there would still be cumbersome or time-limited enrollment processes and information gaps in some states that deter people from signing up, as happens in Medicaid and as we saw in the Children's Health Insurance Program example in chapter 6.

CAN EMPLOYER-SPONSORED INSURANCE DO MORE?

The ACA was built to fill in the gaps between employer-sponsored insurance and government programs. Some may ask why we don't look to employers to close the coverage gap in places where the ACA fell short, since most uninsured people are employed. The problem is that many employers, especially small businesses and those with lower wage structures, do not have the capacity to offer their employees affordable health coverage. For this and other reasons, I don't think we should be looking to expand employer-sponsored insurance. Not only would that require a government mandate on employers (which they are likely to reject), but employers already have enough to contend with in trying to stay competitive amid the pressures of globalization and other market forces. Solving the healthcare coverage problem shouldn't have to be their central concern or a core competency of theirs.

Instead, we should move toward giving employers more viable options that would take health insurance coverage off their hands. America could then take a broader, society-wide view of investing in people's health for the long term. This is how we'll stay productive and competitive in a global economy. Our citizens need a safety net, and employers should contribute to that, but employers should not have to build it or purchase the healthcare platform directly. I recommend phasing out employer-sponsored insurance over a long period of time by providing a worthy public sector-based alternative that incorporates some private sector elements and, over time, shrinks most employers' roles to offering supplemental health benefits. This will help to address issues like job lock, and it will improve employers' competitiveness in the global economy.

G ETTING TO UNIVERSAL COVERAGE will require a holistic approach. In addition to expanding and stitching together a few of the coverage patches (for example, by strengthening the ACA and adopting a reasonable public program expansion proposal), we need a fleece blanket, meaning a fallback public coverage plan for people who don't enroll, which would be paid for by a combination of taxes and premiums. We also need to do things like make enrollment in such a public coverage program automatic, starting with children; this would close the enrollment gaps we see in the CHIP and Medicaid programs. This fleece blanket coverage solution can be basic, but it shouldn't be nothing. We should not leave people out in the cold.

We must also address the threadbare pieces of our coverage quilt, places where people are underinsured. Proposals to strengthen the ACA and create public option programs (like Medicare buy-in) would achieve this by increasing subsidies and capping cost-sharing components in a way that is more generous than the ACA has been to date.

From ideas to implementation, there are many ways to get to universal coverage. It's clear that a hybrid approach, with government and private sector elements, can work. We need more government involvement, but we don't need to go all the way to single-payer. We can take incremental steps, by expanding the pieces of the coverage quilt and stitching in some new ones. History shows us that most Americans prefer an incremental approach. And even though that can be frustratingly slow, it's also more likely to stick.

First, let's be bold and commit to making healthcare a right. Then, we can implement a program, or combination of programs, to make it real. If we commit boldly to making healthcare a right, we can get there, one step at a time. An incremental approach runs the risk of continuing gaps and bare spots, but those can be closed over time, something other countries have done.

In the next chapter, I'll look at how getting to universal coverage aligns with our core values and examine what's feasible—politically, operationally, and financially.

CHAPTER 11

MAKING HEALTHCARE A RIGHT IN THE US

I'm no longer accepting the things I cannot change. I'm changing the things I cannot accept.

—ANGELA DAVIS, feminist activist[1]

THE CHANTS OF "Healthcare is a human right" have echoed in my mind long after the marches were over. The fervor of the deeply felt chants moved me and sparked my interest in figuring out what "making healthcare a right" really means. Other countries treat healthcare as a right. Why not America?

At its core, a country's healthcare system reflects its culture and values. Pew surveys show that "Americans tend to prioritize individual liberty, while Europeans tend to value the role of the state to ensure no one in society is in need."[2] And yet, when Americans have chosen to implement large social programs in the past, including ones that turn certain benefits into rights (such as Social Security and Medicare), they have grown to accept, protect, and even expand them. These programs become part of the social fabric.

How can we do the same with universal healthcare? Embedded in America's founding documents are strongly worded calls for our rights and freedoms. The Declaration of Independence asserts our "unalienable rights," including "life, liberty, and the pursuit of happiness." To this day, Americans place a strong emphasis on the notion of *liberty*, which is often interpreted very individualistically—the freedom to do what we want. But just as important are these words: "All men are created equal" (which in today's world would include women). The ideal of *equality* is also embedded in our society.

The values of liberty and equality are expressed through our political system of democracy and our economic system of free markets and capitalism.

The ways these values are interpreted and prioritized vary tremendously, and that push and pull is at the root of our often-polarized politics. The challenge for Americans is to avoid the extremes. For instance, an extreme version of liberty conjures images of rugged individualism (think cowboys and pioneers), small government, and low taxes. Meanwhile, the extreme version of equality might invoke images of group solidarity, large government, and high taxes. Holding onto extremes like these prevents us from making healthcare a right. Instead, we need to adopt a less individualistic, more interconnected, community-based view that takes a variety of identities, backgrounds, and points-of-view into account with the goal of supporting the common good. Such a view ties back to the principle of shared responsibility embedded in the ACA and can strengthen our social fabric while improving people's individual circumstances.

In a culture that promotes rugged individualism, the prevailing view is that success and failure are entirely determined by the individual, which means that people don't need assistance from a community or government and therefore collective action isn't necessary. Rugged individualism invokes powerful imagery and a mythology (with "macho male" undercurrents) that takes on a life of its own. Rugged individualists have an aversion to redistributing wealth or expanding government's role (actions that get labeled, often incorrectly, "socialism").

But rugged individualism only gets you so far. Rugged individualism didn't land a person on the moon, nor did it build one of the world's best education systems. It also can't raise our nation's children nor care for its elderly. America's greatest achievements have been the result of intense collaboration, combined with intense competition. We are at our best when we keep these things in balance: we need strong communities *and* strong individuals.

Communities are where collaboration happens. The historical roots are deep—early American settlers banded together to build their towns and protect one another. Then, when the thirteen colonies joined to form the United States of America, they chose a community-oriented motto which stands to this day: *E pluribus unum—out of many, one*. Families are also communities, and part of larger communities, as mine has been in Somerville. As a parent, I've experienced the strength of community and collaboration, and I've learned that "it takes a village," not rugged individualism, for children to thrive. Similarly, when I helped lead the launch of health reform in Massachusetts, we were successful because of the strong team that we built and the collaborative way we worked with the community of stakeholders that we served.

That's how I know that it will take community and collaboration to get us to universal healthcare. And government has to be part of the solution: government protects our collective interests (the common good), in addition to our individual rights. This concept of government involvement to support the common good is already embedded in another one of our founding documents, the US Constitution: "The Congress shall have power to lay and collect taxes . . . to provide for the common defense and *general welfare* of the United States" (emphasis mine).

A right to healthcare is certainly consistent with our national values as expressed in these founding documents. The *general welfare* can be interpreted as our population's overall health. And *life* is already defined as an inalienable right in the Declaration of Independence. This can be interpreted as supporting a right to health (without health, there is no life).

Interestingly, protecting some of our other values, such as liberty, already requires a strong government and the taxes to pay for it. We make large public investments for these values: in national defense, to protect our freedom and security, and in our roads and infrastructure, to support our free-market system.

Polls show that many conservatives in the US support the idea of government helping with jobs, healthcare, education, and more. (For example, 90 percent of Republicans and those who lean Republican do not support making cuts to Social Security.)[3] So while Americans may have less egalitarian views than those Europeans hold, public opinion isn't necessarily the obstacle to more egalitarian policies. The public is willing to allocate taxes to popular programs. The key is to figure out what makes a program popular, and then design one in a way that includes those elements.

Based on my experience with implementing health reform over the past fifteen years, one thing is very clear: free markets are an important core value that must be included in any universal healthcare design. That said, they must be tempered.

Throughout this book I've explained market failures and discussed the need for government involvement to deliver universal healthcare. Getting government involved, however, is easier said than done. Free markets (and capitalism) are deeply rooted in our culture—they manifest our value of individual liberty. Americans perceive free markets as being closely linked to democracy, with the same status as freedom of religion, assembly, or speech.

This market frame is so pervasive, it's almost invisible—and it's taken for granted. But it can distort our other frames, such as our views of equality and morality, and of what's fair.

A free-market system certainly brings many positives: it generates innovation, wealth, and some forms of freedom. But as political scientists James Morone and Lawrence Jacobs write, it does not educate everyone's children, conquer segregation, or treat all of those who are sick.[4] As they pointed out, markets are, in fact, powerful engines of inequality. These inequalities are manifested in many ways, including in health disparities, and they cause even more tension between our values of liberty and equality. Adherents to the free-market system prioritize liberty over equality. In fact, as political scientist Deborah Stone says, "(Free) market ideology turns the health care system into a competition between the rich and poor instead of an orderly distribution of medical care according to *medical need*."[5] (Emphasis mine) People who are well-off tend to like markets because they benefit from them. In the case of healthcare coverage, that's a very myopic view, removed from the on-the-ground reality of un- and underinsured people.

To make healthcare a right, we have to temper our current free-market approach to coverage. Achieving meaningful reform and expansion of healthcare coverage requires us to take into account our other social values, like fairness, community, and equal opportunity. In fact, I'm encouraged by the perspective of some feminist economists who have sought to change our frame of reference about classical economics and free markets in several ways, including by taking into consideration our human tendencies toward collaboration (not just competition) and altruism (not just personal gain).[6]

Modern capitalism has been called a "great storm of creative destruction," and that storm has become even more damaging with globalization. We need to buffer our citizens from the storm by reining in the market's excesses. Indeed, as we saw in chapter 4, placing too much reliance on the free market for employer-sponsored health insurance has become increasingly risky. American workers, compared to European ones, are more dependent on their employers for benefits, and women are especially vulnerable since they earn less than men and provide countless hours of unpaid care that don't provide health coverage. Overreliance on the market is also unfair: the majority of uninsured people work and pay taxes that don't give them the health benefits that others are getting. So, while employer-sponsored coverage fits some of our values, such as our affinity for market principles, it does not promote equality, nor does it serve the common good.

There's another health-related problem with unfettered free markets in the global economy: rising inequality. As discussed in chapter 7, inequality is hitting crisis levels. The increasing social distance between rich and poor is hurting our population's health. Policies that reduce income inequalities and strengthen public infrastructure (such as public transport and amenities, public education, public health, and social welfare) are good for population health, but government tends to invest less in them when inequality grows.[7]

And yet, we are often blind to the inequities that exist. We, as Americans, get stuck in a values mind-set in which we believe that our destiny is determined not by our birth, but by our individual abilities and efforts. We believe that we are a meritocracy that provides equal opportunity: so strong are our myth-like beliefs in equality and social mobility that we don't see the fact we have erected tremendous systemic barriers to upward mobility. And that's damaging. Because of this meritocracy myth, we tolerate inequality more than people in other countries do, and it's affecting our health.

We talk about individuals needing to make healthy choices, but it's difficult to do so in a toxic environment of inequality. While a handful of Jeff Bezos–types control an extraordinary amount of wealth, most Americans are struggling to make ends meet. Forty percent of Americans couldn't cover an unexpected expense of four hundred dollars, which is far less than most health insurance deductibles.[8] Individual choices are important, but they are always made in the broader context of an environment we don't control. And inequality leads to premature deaths. As noted previously, uninsured and underinsured people get less care and they get it later in illness episodes because they defer treatment. T. R. Reid sums it up well when he says, "In the US, the well-off get the best medical care in the world, and people in the bottom brackets get so little care that thousands die of treatable diseases."[9] My own cancer treatment is a perfect example of the well-off end of this spectrum: as nerve-wracking as it all was, I had the relative peace of mind that came from having great health insurance coverage and great care. I benefited from early detection, from an extra MRI test to confirm the recommended treatment, and from immediate surgery with the most advanced techniques. As a result, I never had to tell my kids that I might die. People who have to defer treatment will not be as fortunate.

Tackling inequality will require opening our eyes to these unacceptable, unhealthy extremes and then taking action to temper markets and redistribute income and benefits. Universal healthcare is one way to do this. The first step is to make it a right.

AMERICAN VALUES SUPPORT MAKING HEALTHCARE A RIGHT

As I've dug deeper into figuring out why healthcare is not yet a right in America, I've come to realize that many people just aren't aware of how bad life is without decent health insurance. It is also now clear to me that since our healthcare coverage "system" (if you can call it that) evolved in such a piecemeal fashion that we never really had an opportunity to debate the "healthcare is a right" question as a society. As Reid writes in *The Healing of America*, there was "no serious assessment of national values."[10] He goes on to say that the primary decision about making healthcare a right is a moral one, and I agree.

It's a moral imperative to make healthcare a right for all US citizens. Healthcare is a human right, which means it's a right that exists independent of our culture, religion, race, nationality, or economic status. Health is foundational to our lives. Without our health we—literally—cannot live, let alone live with dignity. We can't enjoy any other rights without it.

There is also a democratic imperative. Polls show that universal healthcare is what Americans want, so enacting such a program would be responsive to popular preference—a good thing in a democracy. And, importantly, when healthcare coverage is only a privilege for the advantaged, we undermine our collective sense of basic social equality. As inequalities become more extreme and locked in, our sense of full community membership is also undermined.[11] The result: people are less likely to participate in our democracy. Healthy citizens participate more fully, from staying informed, to volunteering, to voting. It's similar to having educated citizens (one of the benefits of making K–12 education a right). There's an interdependence between social mobility and democracy—social mobility is a common good that benefits our society.

Plus, there's an economic imperative that's related to fairness. Basic health is necessary for a genuine meritocracy. Fair competition necessitates equality of opportunity, which means we need education, food, and decent housing, and access to healthcare. Moreover, universal healthcare is a human capital investment that will improve our economic competitiveness as a country—it benefits our current and future workforce and allows people to be far more productive. And it's a virtuous circle: healthy people are more likely to invest in their own education and job skills, which enhances the value of society's investment in universal healthcare.

On a related note, countries with universal healthcare have more of an incentive to keep people healthy over the years, because they ultimately share the same risk pool. One of government's jobs is to protect people, and it helps if there's an economic incentive to do so. In the US' fragmented healthcare system, economic incentives for preventive care are dissipated, in large part because the average person with health insurance stays with the same plan for fewer than six years.[12] Contrast that with Britain's National Health Service, where people are patients for life.

Finally, the US is an outlier on the international stage. As a wealthy nation, it's especially shameful that we haven't yet found a way to make healthcare a right. Most wealthy nations have done so, and they have also found ways to protect their citizens from the extreme effects of global competition.[13] In 1966, the United Nations adopted a treaty for its member nations to pursue universal coverage, Article 12 of which says "states must protect this right [to physical and mental health] through a comprehensive system of healthcare which is available to everyone without discrimination and economically accessible to all." *It was ratified by every country except three: Palau, Comoros, and the United States.*[14]

In sum, our society can't be harmonious or fully productive if we leave people uncovered and out in the cold. Severe inequalities of income and wealth damage our sense of national community, contribute to crime, undermine the ideal of equal opportunity, and decrease the aggregate welfare of Americans.[15] Nobel Prize–winning economist Paul Krugman captured it well: "The simple fact is that there is far more misery in America than there needs to be."[16]

AMERICA IS MORE than just a collection of rugged individualists pursuing personal freedoms and self-interest. Americans have realized the limits of individualism and turned to government in times of crisis. As President Franklin D. Roosevelt famously stated in 1933 during the Great Depression, "We now realize as we have never realized before our interdependence on one another." Likewise, Dr. Martin Luther King Jr. wrote about interdependence in 1963 in his "Letter from a Birmingham Jail":

> Injustice anywhere is a threat to justice everywhere. We are caught in an inescapable network of mutuality, tied in a single garment of destiny. Whatever affects one directly, affects all indirectly. . . . Anyone who lives inside the United States can never be considered an outsider anywhere within its bounds.[17]

President Roosevelt set the stage for making healthcare a right in his 1941 State of the Union address, in which he defined "four essential human freedoms," including freedom from want. He then called for a second Bill of Rights in his 1944 State of the Union address, including "the right to medical care and the opportunity to achieve and enjoy good health."

Even though Roosevelt didn't achieve universal healthcare during his lifetime, these values were carried forward by subsequent presidents, including Harry Truman, John F. Kennedy, Lyndon Johnson, and Barack Obama. We ended up with more patches in the coverage quilt as a result, including Medicare, Medicaid, and the ACA.

Since many of America's leaders have supported making healthcare a right, it's only natural to have questions about what that really means. Author and surgeon Atul Gawande recently chronicled his conversations about healthcare with his former high school classmates in a small town in Ohio, and they were clear about their concerns. As much as they needed healthcare, they couldn't see making healthcare a right without also making it a responsibility. Otherwise, it might undermine people's work efforts, they said. In addition, they recognized that "one person's right to healthcare becomes another person's burden to pay for it." Gawande's classmates argued that they didn't want to pay taxes to help people who "don't deserve it."[18]

These concerns point to several other prevailing notions of our culture, including our strong work ethic. Closely tied to our values of individualism and free markets, our work ethic translates into moral judgments regarding who is succeeding or failing in our society. This, in turn, fuels our determinations about who is "deserving" versus "undeserving" of government-sponsored benefit programs. Many Americans are quick to assume that people who receive government-funded benefits are not working or are lazy (unless it's Social Security or Medicare, in which case people "paid in" and now "deserve" their benefits).

That said, ongoing genetic research is showing us that there are fewer areas than previously believed where illness is a person's "fault." Recognizing there is a genetic lottery at birth helps to reduce the strength of the deserving/undeserving frame of reference. In addition, most of the uninsured and underinsured are working people. They are proud and don't want to be perceived as taking a "handout." They want to be part of the system with decent insurance coverage that everyone else is in, and they are willing to pay in what they can afford.

In short, we can't talk about rights in America without matching them with responsibilities. As Gawande points out, "Rights are as much about our duties as about our freedoms."[19] This was vividly on display recently when

I attended a military gathering with my son, who is in Army ROTC. As we cheered the racing soldiers on, I was struck by the words on one soldier's sign: "Freedom isn't free." The men and women of our armed forces certainly know the meaning of duty and the price of freedom. As Americans, we should all be proud to accept certain responsibilities. And healthcare as a right should be one of them.

Making healthcare a right in the US requires balancing individual freedom with our responsibility to support the common good. It means turning "individual freedom versus collective responsibility" into a "both-and" rather than an "either-or" issue, as public health experts Elizabeth Bradley and Lauren Taylor write in *The American Health Care Paradox*.[20] This balance embraces shared responsibility, as embodied in the ACA's three-legged stool framework. The ACA was unique because it made coverage both an entitlement and a responsibility of citizenship. In so doing, it advanced the idea of making healthcare a right—of having universal healthcare for the *whole* population, not just a subset by age or income.

So now is the time to ask the question: Do we want to make healthcare a right, like education? Or keep it as a commodity, like a car? Making healthcare a right is consistent with our national values. In fact, it can be viewed as a patriotic act—one that protects our citizens and serves our country.

Our universal healthcare solution needs to reward work while protecting those who are vulnerable. It also needs to balance individual with community interests, and freedom with responsibility. To those ends, the universal healthcare solution must include these core principles:

- Be truly universal (cover everyone)—this will be perceived as fair and ensure the broadest base of support.
- Achieve a balance between rights and responsibilities—we should view this as a pact with our government, rather than a mandate.
- Contain some elements of the free market, like consumer choice and innovation—this supports the value of individual freedom.
- Be something people pay into, like Social Security or Medicare, so that it's perceived as an "earned benefit"—this supports the values of hard work and responsibility and helps us to move away from the "deserving/undeserving" beneficiary trap.
- Ensure access to quality care for all and make the benefits affordable via a sliding scale of payments (based on income)—this will address inequality.

PATH TO A SOLUTION

In the US, rights can be established in many ways. Some rights are enshrined in the Constitution (like the Bill of Rights), some are embedded in a law (like the Social Security Act), and some are established by the courts. The Supreme Court views the right to healthcare as a political process issue, which means legislation is needed. Even though the Fourteenth Amendment of the Constitution contains a right to liberty, the Supreme Court won't interpret it more broadly to mean a right to healthcare.[21]

Rights can also take different forms. Some are political (such as one person, one vote) and some are social (such as government programs that provide services or cash assistance to provide a basic standard of living or make human capital investments). People are more likely to use their political rights if they are benefiting from social rights (since they have protections they don't want to lose)—this is certainly true in the case of seniors, with Medicare and Social Security.

In terms of which legislative path to pursue, federal legislation is more feasible than seeking an amendment to the US Constitution. It's unlikely that we'll get a constitutional amendment for a right to healthcare; we still haven't managed to adopt the Equal Rights Amendment of 1972, which would simply state that women and men are guaranteed equal legal rights. With that in mind, it's most expedient to push for national legislation that can be passed by Congress and signed by the president.

Establishing a right to healthcare means that society would have an obligation to provide it. So it's more than just getting a law passed. For the right to be *real*, the legislation will have to include a well-designed program with an enforcement mechanism attached to it, as well as a source of funds. This is how K–12 education and entitlement programs like Social Security and Medicare work. There's a long distance to travel from political rhetoric to policy reality. As the old saying goes, "talk is cheap." It's one thing to say that healthcare should be a right, and another thing entirely to design, implement, and fund a program that works.

There *is* a path to universal healthcare that can work for Americans. There are elements of proposals in chapter 10 that can be combined and that will work. However it's designed, the solution needs to be simple for people to understand and sustainable, both politically and economically. And it needs to start with where we are today. To a large extent, we are beholden to the healthcare and coverage system we already have—this is the notion of "path dependency," in which existing systems are too hard to undo, and therefore shape the "parameters of the possible." We simply can't start from scratch—it would be far too difficult and very disruptive.

Indeed, the US has made healthcare a right for some already: the elderly, most of the poor, and those with severe emergency care needs (defined as severe risk of death or in active labor, until stabilized). Many mistakenly believe that the US has a fully privatized healthcare system, and yet we are already "semi-socialized" (meaning partially government-run) for almost half of our healthcare system. The proposals for universal healthcare, such as Medicare for All and the Medicare buy-in options, reflect these realities; as discussed in chapter 10, they build on what Americans like that is already working.

This policy design process should include identifying the sources of funding for universal healthcare, as well as an implementation plan. The latter is beyond the scope of this book, but suffice it to say that since many people don't entirely trust government, we need to go slowly with implementation, making it a multiyear process, and build credibility for universal healthcare along the way.

FUNDING

As for funding, some will say that given the current level of healthcare spending and its high rate of growth, we can't afford universal healthcare. It's a valid concern. Indeed, current spending on healthcare is crowding out a great deal of other spending in the public sector (for education and other necessary public goods) and at the household level: the premiums for family coverage cost more than a mortgage payment, and the premiums for individual coverage cost more than a car payment. We should be asking ourselves why we aren't getting a better return on investment for the money we are already spending. We cannot ignore how poorly we are performing relative to other wealthy nations.

Universal coverage is actually more affordable in other countries—they don't spend as much per person on healthcare as the US does. This is because their governments regulate healthcare prices to keep them in check. These countries also make wise, health-improving investments beyond universal coverage: they spend more (relatively) on prevention and social services than the US does.

But it's not just about the absolute cost of healthcare or how funds are invested. It's also about the available funding. One of the biggest obstacles to enacting universal coverage in the US is the *perceived* lack of funding. But there are plenty of potential funding approaches. In fact, there's enough money to fund universal coverage. The dollars that are available for health-care spending relate back to what a society values. Some dollars will need to be reallocated, which will be contentious. It's ultimately a question of priorities. Other countries believe they can't afford *not* to invest in universal coverage. The US should—and can—follow their lead.

How much money is needed for universal healthcare depends on which solution we decide to pursue. In chapter 10, I described what an extremely generous single-payer program like Medicare for All might cost: an average of $4 trillion per year over a ten-year period (it will start lower and end higher over that period). That high price tag is going to generate extreme sticker shock for most Americans, especially if it has to be funded by taxes. Fortunately, there are less expensive approaches that can be taken.

For example, if we took *incremental coverage expansion and affordability steps* instead, and left the employer-sponsored insurance system alone, we won't have to find as much money. That sounds good to me. Here's a back-of-the envelope calculation:

1. Cover twenty-eight million uninsured people @ $6,000/year (average premium) = *$168 billion per year*
2. Add to that some funds to help cover out-of-pocket costs for those with commercial insurance, on a sliding scale basis. Assume an average of $1,000 x 180 million people = *$180 billion per year*.
3. TOTAL of 1 + 2: Approximately *$350 billion per year*

The total of $350 billion—that's about 10 percent of our current $3.65 trillion spending on healthcare. It sounds like a lot of money, but it can be found. There are three main areas we can look. We can (1) find savings within the healthcare system, (2) raise revenues, and (3) reduce spending for current programs. Within each of these categories, there are many, many ideas that could be pursued. Think of these ideas as potential building blocks that could be put together in different ways. Applying a shared responsibility approach would mean that we take some from each category. The bottom line is that even just a few of these ideas would more than cover expanded healthcare coverage in the US.

For starters, there are many terrific ideas for how to obtain savings in the healthcare system itself. The Institute of Medicine found that the US wastes $750 billion every year on medical care, including $340 billion in unnecessary or inefficiently delivered services.[22] While it's tough to carve out waste that is marbled into the system, surely we could find more efficiencies. For example, having a back surgery when a less invasive, less expensive treatment would have worked just as well is waste. Some of the waste is administrative costs. A General Accounting Office report found that if the US was able to get its healthcare administrative costs to the Canadian level, we would save enough money to cover all of the uninsured people in the country (forty-five million people, at the time the study was conducted).[23] Speaking of Canada, if we could pay what the Canadians pay for their pharmaceuticals, we could save at least $100 billion per year—clearly there's an opportunity to negotiate better drug prices.[24]

Another idea is to regulate the prices of healthcare providers (doctors and hospitals) as other countries do and as the US does for Medicare and Medicaid. If all commercially covered healthcare was paid at Medicare provider rates, the system would save $400 billion per year.[25] While that may be too draconian, changing even a portion would help. And finally, we should invest more in prevention: in the US, more money is spent on curing disease than on preventing it and promoting healthy behaviors. We need to shift the balance, both within our healthcare spending and to more social services spending.

The next category is finding ways of raising revenues to fund universal healthcare, and there is plenty of opportunity. In fact, we can raise revenues in a way that will decrease inequality. The US has the lowest individual tax rates of any industrialized nation, particularly on its top earners.[26] The 2017 tax cuts are further exacerbating the already deep inequalities in wealth we have today. Undoing these tax cuts would save the government about $200 billion per year. Similarly, the 2017 corporate tax cuts could be restored, and raise $140 billion per year.

We could also implement a small, Medicare-like payroll tax to cover some costs. Americans are used to the idea of funding their future Medicare benefits this way. Psychologically, connecting the Medicare payment with payroll makes it almost like paying a health insurance premium, rather than paying a tax. Another option is reducing the $250 billion tax break for employer-sponsored insurance or making it more progressive. In addition, we could tax unhealthy items, like sugary drinks, and raise taxes on cigarettes and alcohol—this would have the added benefit of reducing our healthcare spending.

Lastly, there are many federal programs with funds that could be redeployed to support universal healthcare. The first two I would target are the excess spending on defense and prisons. We need to rebalance this spending to better promote our collective health and well-being. Every year the US spends about $600 billion to $750 billion on defense.[27] That's more than the total spent by the next *eight* countries combined! Efficiencies could be found at the US Pentagon; one report estimates we could save $125 billion there, and we could also buy less equipment and save billions of dollars.[28] As for our prisons: we spend over $180 billion every year on incarceration, and one in five inmates, or half a million people, are in jail for nonviolent drug offenses.[29] If these nonviolent inmates were sent to treatment, rather than jail, we'd save at least $30 billion per year. Bottom line: we should be far more concerned about the threats to our lives from our lack of universal healthcare than a military threat from another country or dangers from nonviolent drug offenders.

Choosing among these options should be based on the principles of balance and fairness that were embodied in the ACA's three-legged stool approach, which combines individual responsibility with corporate and government contributions. In addition, a program as extensive as universal healthcare needs to be sustainably funded. It's best to diversify risk by taking an approach that doesn't rely too heavily on any one source of funds or savings. This also makes things fairer politically. Such an approach should be positioned for the upside if there's economic growth (meaning more revenue without tax increases).

To be fiscally sustainable, the universal healthcare solution also has to have mechanisms embedded in it that obtain savings in the healthcare system. The healthcare system has become very overweight and is crowding out funding for other important investments. We need to put the system on a "diet" through some combination of price regulation and global budgeting. This approach can work for a single-payer or multipayer solution. It needs to be done in a smart way: paying lower prices is necessary to make universal healthcare affordable, but it doesn't guarantee better health outcomes—it just means that we spend less for certain things. There need to be incentives to ensure that we are spending on the right things, and not too many things.

Some funding solutions will be contentious. That said, while taxes are never popular, some are perceived by the general population as "less evil" than others, like the so-called sin taxes on cigarettes and unhealthy food. Raising taxes that help to mitigate the extreme level of inequality in the US is an issue that will resonate for many potential voters and activists.

Bringing some of the "hidden" ways that we currently pay for healthcare (such as the tax deduction for employer-sponsored insurance) explicitly onto the federal budget and raising taxes to pay for it, as some Medicare for All proposals do, would be a big challenge, given Americans' dislike of taxes. A more palatable approach would be the way Social Security and Medicare were originally set up, with people paying into a trust fund dedicated to that purpose, and from which they draw benefits later.

It's ultimately a question of priorities, and those priorities can be influenced by our political activism. Other countries believe they can't afford *not* to invest in universal coverage. Let's get the US to follow their lead.

CREATING POLITICAL WILL

The key to getting to universal healthcare is developing the political will. As Morone writes, "Political wills find fiscal ways."[30] Remember, we are a wealthy country. We can make the case to the general public that universal healthcare is worth paying for. It starts with raising awareness. We need to share compelling stories and deliver clear, hard-hitting messages.

Fortunately, increasing numbers of people, and especially millennials, are realizing how tenuous their grip is on the current system of health coverage. Call it "enlightened self-interest," but there's an increasing interest in finding ways to cover benefits *outside* of the employer-based system. They are seeking a more compassionate version of capitalism. They are ready to hear these proposals. We need to make sure they have that chance.

Some countries, like England after World War II, were able to build their healthcare systems virtually from scratch. The US, on the other hand, does not need to rebuild after catastrophic devastation, and it has a very entrenched healthcare system full of vested interests (doctors, insurers, hospital boards) that are bound to push back on anything perceived as detrimental. So, is change even possible? It is.

Just look at what other countries have done. Both Taiwan and Switzerland redesigned their healthcare systems relatively recently (in the early 1990s) to guarantee universal health coverage. Both countries have been described as "ferociously capitalistic" with "vigorous democracies" (they have political parties that are similar to ours). Each country was able to work through some tough politics, including entrenched political and business interests and opposing philosophical approaches to government.[31] Still, they studied what other countries had done, and they found ways to apply those lessons to their systems. Advocates and the liberal parties increased the pressure for change so much that conservatives chose not to resist. Advocates focused more on the moral issue than the details of the reform plans, stressing that society had an ethical obligation to implement the changes.[32]

None of the systems that other countries have adopted is perfect. But we can't let the perfect be the enemy of the good—change is desperately needed. We also have to recognize that health reform is an ongoing process, not an end state. We need a bold vision, one that can be realized through incremental, digestible steps. And there will need to be some compromise.

To get there, we have to open up our hearts and minds. It will require a broader view of what's possible than many of us have. We need to think about health as a shared responsibility for our larger community, not just a result of our "individual choices and failings." This will help us to address the social determinants of health, which, as Bradley and Taylor pointed out, "are best addressed through collective action."[33] We may not be comfortable with this, but as I've been emphasizing, we are interrelated and interdependent with those with whom we share a common pool of resources. As Dr. Martin Luther King Jr. said, "All life is interrelated. The agony of the poor impoverishes the rich; the betterment of the poor enriches the rich. We are inevitably our brother's keeper because we are our brother's brother. Whatever affects one directly affects all indirectly."[34]

W E CAN AND MUST move from the rhetoric to the reality of making healthcare a right in America. The reasons can be summed up in four parts:

1. It's a moral imperative.
2. It aligns with our values.
3. There are feasible solutions that fit our culture.
4. We can fund it.

And it's not too late!

It all boils down to our priorities. In a wealthy country, the ability to fund something comes down to priorities, not resources. Compared to other wealthy countries, *we are the least taxed, most armed, and most unequal country*. Our health outcomes reflect this reality. We lag behind other nations on the basics, and frankly it's embarrassing.

We can do better. A total of twenty-six thousand people die each year because they don't have health insurance. Our spending and taxation approaches reflect our priorities, and we have a lot of room for improvement. Universal healthcare is an investment we should be making. We can't afford not to. We had a crisis with the Great Recession of 2008, and given the inevitability of economic cycles, there will be another one. We are already facing a crisis of increasing inequality in our country, advancing at a meteoric rate. Millions of workers are being disrupted by the global economy, and that trend is here to stay. Families are facing a crisis at their kitchen tables as they juggle bills and are forced to choose between making a housing payment or a deductible payment to get needed healthcare. In the midst of these crises, we must demand social change.

It's not necessary to become a policy expert and master the details of our legislative system in order to fix it—that can be left to the professionals. The key is to create a mandate for change so that healthcare becomes a right in the US. Moving to universal healthcare is possible—it will take moral imagination and courageous empathy.[35] We simply have to develop the political will.

CHAPTER 12

. . . . . .

THE ACTIVISM AGENDA

To bring about change, you must not be afraid to take the first step.
We will fail when we fail to try.

—ROSA PARKS, civil rights activist[1]

T HE CHANTS FROM THE MARCHES AND RALLIES I've attended continue to
reverberate. In addition to "Healthcare is a human right!" I hear, "Tell
me what democracy looks like—this is what democracy looks like!" These
moments are powerful and full of potential. And so are women.

It's time for us to join together and rally to make healthcare a right. Our
patchwork quilt of health coverage is threadbare and full of holes. We can fix
it: we have tremendous potential power and we can ignite a social movement
for universal healthcare.

Our moral outrage can drive change. With it, we can fuel a social movement, create the political will, and harness the power to overcome the status
quo, including the entrenched interests of industry participants.

Social movements are aspirational. They require big ideas, energetic
leadership, and widespread participation. We have to excite the passion for a
social movement. We need to dwell in possibility. As political scientist Marie
Gottschalk writes, "Much of politics is about developing a new vision that
transcends the given political environment . . . and ultimately transforms
[it]."[2] Bold activism around making healthcare a right will change our culture and make universal healthcare a political imperative.

We don't have to define the detailed policy solutions—political situations are always fluid, so it's impossible to identify in advance all the details
of solutions, nor can we predict the exact timing of success. Instead, we need
to get the attention of politicians and the media. We need to help create
"windows of opportunity" to move solutions forward. The policy experts
can work with interest groups and others to develop the details.

And we have to persist. We have to overcome the inertia that is built into American politics. It's possible, if we embrace the same spirit that Speaker Nancy Pelosi brought to the fight to pass the ACA. As she said at the time:

> We will go through the gate. If the gate is closed, we will go over the fence. If the fence is too high, we will pole-vault in. If that doesn't work, we will parachute in. But we are going to get health reform passed.[3]

In this way, our discontent can be turned into legislative victories.

WOMEN SHOULD LEAD THE WAY

The path to universal coverage will require our collective participation and activism. To rally support, we need to include those who have a strong personal stake in the issue. That's why women should lead the way. Whether we realize it or not, every woman has a personal stake in this issue. Healthcare for all is more than a good idea; it's a necessary facet of a truly just society.

It's time to turn the personal into the political because so many of us need these healthcare coverage issues to be solved. These are universal problems that require a universal solution. Free-market failures won't cure themselves—it takes political will to get government to act.

In chapter 8, I showed how women's voting patterns reflect the fact that many of us already prioritize healthcare as an issue, and that there's bipartisan common ground around our concerns about the affordability of healthcare. These voting patterns show that mobilizing women is key to enacting universal healthcare: we need to encourage all candidates to support universal coverage proposals, particularly ones that address healthcare costs, and then get more women out to vote.

Women continually rank healthcare as a top priority because women tend to carry the burden of figuring out healthcare for their families. Women are disproportionately tasked with the emotional labor required to keep a family healthy and functioning—watching and worrying over sick children, caring for parents and friends, remembering to schedule medical appointments and find ways to get everyone to the right place on time, remembering to pay the medical bills—even deciding whether to see a specialist or try a cheaper remedy for a sprained knee or a lingering cold. This kind of care, though necessary, is not as easily quantifiable as the time spent in professional roles. Emotional labor goes above and beyond what's measurable, contributing to the stress that women face every day. It's wrapped around the 80 percent of all healthcare decisions that women make in the home, and it amps up when we are forced to confront issues we can't solve on our own, such as an unexpected spike in insurance premiums or loss of coverage for a preexisting condition. All of this stress is compounded by the fact that women often take personal responsibility for systemic societal problems that, particularly in the context of healthcare, can increase our feelings of helplessness and lead to emotional burnout.

That's what happened to me in late 2017. My "last straw" moment came a few months after my breast cancer surgery, while I was coping with my own recovery, managing care for my aging parents, and trying to help my daughter adjust to her new celiac diagnosis from three thousand miles away. At the same time, I was juggling multiple stressors at work, and the #MeToo movement was hitting a crescendo, adding to the deeply upsetting national debates already happening around ACA repeal and other issues related to social justice and equality. I was overburdened emotionally, but I didn't know it until a family member asked me to organize a family gathering—a request that I would have, under other circumstances, taken in stride. Instead, I broke down—not in that moment, but days later, when I finally shared my feelings with my husband. "This is all just too much," I remember telling him. "I'm completely maxed out and I don't know what more I can do." I was on a path to burnout.

For me, activism is a salve. When I get involved with others in creating positive change, I feel less burdened with the heavy lifting of emotional labor and the stress of systemic issues that seem so hard to change. As activist and author Grace Lee Boggs said, "Building community is to the collective as spiritual practice is to the individual."[4] It reminds me of what one doctor in training said: "To fight burnout, *we should never worry alone* about the social determinants of health that patients face. *To fight burnout, organize.*"[5] (Emphasis mine.)

One of the most compelling things I've learned about activism is that it not only helps the cause you're working on, it also helps you as an individual by adding meaning to your life, offering a group to belong to and people to connect with, and serving as an outlet for frustration. It helps you grow intellectually and emotionally. Three of my heroes, Angela Davis, Cecile Richards, and Gloria Steinem, have talked extensively about the personal benefits of activism.[6] Activism can help women feel less alone as they share the burden of caregiving and join forces to advocate for change. That's important, because the lack of healthcare access is a systemic problem, bigger than we are as individuals and families. As a result, it can be especially drain-ing. Steinem summed it up this way: "My mother paid a high price for car-ing so much, yet being able to do so little about it. In this way, she led me toward an activist place where she herself could never go."[7]

Activism can lessen feelings of helplessness and burnout by connect-ing you to a community that's dedicated to meaningful change. This can make you happier and healthier overall. As happiness expert Gretchen Ru-bin writes in her best-selling book, *The Happiness Project*, "Having strong social bonds is probably the *most* meaningful contributor to happiness."[8] Rubin joins many other happiness scholars in advocating for strong inter-personal relationships. Studies show that strong ties to community lengthen life, boost immunity to illness, and decrease risk of depression—and this holds true whether you're an introvert or an extrovert. In addition, advocat-ing for healthcare as a right can be the kind of "challenging fun" that Rubin says helps us develop strong personal bonds, mastery of a skill, and create an atmosphere of growth—all of which further contribute to our overall experience of happiness.

Think of activism as a dynamic continuum of involvement, where your position will change from time to time. There may be days when you feel like being on the front lines, and days when you'll take a quieter, more pri-vate approach. How you engage will also depend on what's needed in the moment. For instance, based on the Personal Activism Assessment I've de-veloped (see my website, https://rosemarieday.com), you may find yourself in the category that is comfortable with sharing stories but feels unready to participate in a public protest. In this case, you could challenge yourself to share more deeply by finding opportunities to have conversations with people beyond your inner circle, to raise their level of awareness and com-mitment to the cause of expanding healthcare coverage. This approach can work in many venues, including corporate America. Debra Meyerson coined the term "tempered radical" to describe people who are making a difference in large companies. "Rather than pressing their agendas, [tempered radicals] start conversations," she writes. "Like steady drops of water, they gradually erode granite."[9] People in this category understand that change takes time, and they are effective because they focus on influencing hearts and minds as the start to impacting policy.

∎ ∎ ∎

YPICALLY, IT'S EASIER to *know* that something needs to be done, rather than to actually *do* something about it, and paradoxically, women are often more in touch with the obstacles we face than with the need for activism. That's because there are several layers of obstacles, including those that are most immediate (such as a lack of time, doubt that you can make a difference, or discomfort with controversy), and those that present longer term, psychological barriers (such as negative stereotypes and social pressures), and structural barriers (such as outright discrimination, including racism and sexism).

The good news is that there are many ways to overcome these challenges, individually and collectively. (See my website, https://rosemarieday.com, for some tips.) A key thing to remember as you step up your activism level is that you are advocating for more than yourself—you are advocating for others as well by pushing for universal healthcare. This can make it easier to ask political leaders for change. It can also be enormously helpful to join advocacy organizations such as Community Catalyst, Families USA, or MomsRising. These organizations find ways to make getting involved as easy as possible. When I spoke with Kristin Rowe-Finkbeiner, the cofounder and CEO of MomsRising, she was clear that lack of time is one of the biggest obstacles that women and moms face, so her organization addresses that in creative ways. For example, MomsRising and other advocacy organizations will clue you in to key times and easy ways to be involved once you sign up for their "action alerts." If you sign up and get too many requests, you can always opt out or change your preferences so that you receive alerts less frequently. And you can always say no if the time isn't right for you.

To address structural barriers to activism, such as sexism, the key is to remember that we have strength in our numbers. By raising our awareness, harnessing our anger and frustrations, and connecting through social media and political action, women can rise up and make change. As feminist journalist and author Rebecca Traister chronicled in *Good and Mad*, "Women's anger spurs creativity and drives innovation in politics and social change—it always has."[10] Working together can be exhilarating. I've experienced the moment of joy Traister describes—the one that happens when you are surrounded by people who feel your same sense of anger and who also want to do something about it. It has happened at all of the Women's Marches and healthcare rallies that I've attended.[11] Pushing for universal healthcare calls for an inclusive and intersectional kind of activism, which makes sense—our collective health impacts many different facets of society.

RALLYING

To improve healthcare coverage in America, we need to rally for universal healthcare. Making healthcare a right in the US has to be our unequivocal goal. In so doing, the key is to (1) always think big, (2) define core principles, (3) negotiate the details, and (4) never stop pushing.

I'll weave these ideas into the next sections as I talk more about what we should rally for. Because as we are thinking big and pushing forward on universal healthcare, we can and should work on other things along the way, including protecting the ACA and advocating for state coverage solutions. We should also address the social determinants of health at both the state and national level.

UNIVERSAL HEALTHCARE

To make healthcare a right in the US, we have to think big and advocate for a universal healthcare solution, ideally one that is politically feasible. That said, we shouldn't get stuck on what's feasible right now—we need to keep focused on what's desirable. We also don't need a perfectly defined solution before an election. We need first to agree on a national goal: *affordable health coverage for all Americans.* This is our most important core principle and should not be negotiated (other core principles are listed in chapter 11).

The key is to think big while taking small steps. Big ideas energize social movements more than small ones do: they mobilize people by capturing their imaginations and giving them hope.[12] Thinking big also helps to prevent backsliding and ensures that the small steps really add up, while positioning us to demand bigger changes if the window of opportunity opens (the timing of which can be very unpredictable, but is more assured if we keep the pressure on). And it's all right to divide our efforts between big causes and small ones as long as we keep the big picture in mind.

As soon as the policy details for universal healthcare begin to take shape, we can expect plenty of opposition. It is easy for opponents to tap into anti-government views with cries of "socialism." And there are many invested in the status quo who lobby and vote: healthcare providers, insurers, business, labor groups, and the elderly. We need to address the opposition, which reflects some core values in our country. In so doing, we need to stick to our core principles, which also reflect our country's core values. We can then allow negotiation of some policy details, but we can leave that to the experts.

It's tempting for policy wonks like me to look for a technical solution to lift the healthcare debate beyond partisanship and politics. This can be helpful, but it doesn't inspire people to act. One of the reasons we don't yet have universal coverage is that many health reform advocates have focused more on developing intricate policy proposals than on winning popular support for their proposals. But if a program is too complex, we can't explain it quickly.

To counter this, we need to create a simple message that invokes the moral imperative, wrapped in a message of patriotism. And politicians have to feel their political lives depend on making healthcare a right. We then have to push this, relentlessly.

We may have to get to universal healthcare in incremental steps. This will require persistence. The same was true for Medicare—it didn't cover everything for seniors when it first started (and it still doesn't, but it's come a long way). I'm a big fan of the practicalities of incrementalism. If small steps are all we can achieve initially, it's much better than nothing. Incrementalism adds up.

ONE THING WORKING IN OUR FAVOR is that there are a lot more people who are likely to rally for universal healthcare now because the threat of a repeal of the ACA caught voters' attention and increased the number of people who are likely to make healthcare a priority when they vote. The ACA brought more people into the conversation because it targeted *everyone*—not just particular subgroups of the population like the elderly or the disabled. The ACA provided *universal* protections, including protections for preexisting conditions. As a result, people are much more in touch with the concept of protecting preexisting conditions now, and they will go to the mat to fight for these protections. They have been galvanized, thanks to the efforts of numerous organizations (such as Families USA, MoveOn.org, and Planned Parenthood), who have shared people's stories and resisted the ACA's repeal efforts. This means there are groups that are ready and eager to fight for more.

We can expand the numbers willing to fight for universal healthcare by including people who don't have immediate healthcare needs but understand and value the needs of others—those with "enlightened preferences." Beyond that, the fragility of the current coverage system, including its ties to jobs in an uncertain economy, should bring more people into the coverage constituency. As healthcare historian Beatrix Hoffman writes, "The workers, seniors, and poor families who were formerly protected by job benefits,

Medicare, and Medicaid now have more in common with the uninsured and the underinsured."[13] I encourage anyone who currently enjoys good healthcare coverage to develop enlightened preferences, and vote not just their immediate self-interest. There's an added urgency for high-income people to join this fight, since they vote at higher rates and make larger political donations.[14]

People can develop enlightened preferences when they have enough information about the issues of others. Ideally, in an inclusive democracy, the issues of others can be brought forward, shared, and discussed. The media can be a powerful source of stories about these issues, as can books and movies. Social media is ideal for amplifying these stories. The key is tapping into emotions and experience, as well as facts. Through this process people can develop a deeper understanding of others' issues and ultimately embrace them as their own desire for universal healthcare.

There are also some new and influential groups we can rally. Unlike in the past, more doctors support the concept of universal healthcare. Their support has been increasing—doctors are frustrated with the myriad insurance bureaucracies they deal with and the issue of uninsured people. In fact, the American Medical Association adopted the position that healthcare is a human right at its annual meeting in June 2019. Younger physicians are more used to the idea of universal healthcare (the American Medical Student Association now supports it). And the number of physicians who are women is growing, and women are more likely to support a mandate for universal healthcare.[15]

In addition, millennials are ripe to rally—they are more likely to support universal healthcare. And we know that the vast majority of uninsured people would prefer to be insured—they just can't afford it.

Next, since we have so many folks we can rally, and we know that 92 percent of the general public supports making healthcare a right, we need to turn that support into action. It starts with building greater awareness and understanding since the actual approach to universal healthcare is less well understood and support for it varies, often depending on the terminology used in the poll; "Medicare for All" is a more popular term than "single-payer," for example.

We then need to communicate the "fierce urgency of now," as Dr. Martin Luther King Jr. invoked during the March on Washington. We should seize moments that create a sense of urgency. Case in point: it was easier to focus people on the imminent threat of ACA repeal in 2017 than to organize a rally for universal coverage. The fear of having something taken away is more immediately powerful than the hope for something people don't yet have.

Gunnar Almgren, a healthcare-as-a-right proponent, writes that the ACA gave a face to the previously unseen people and gave many of us a vision for an alternative future in this country.[16] Each of these faces and stories helps to lay the groundwork for a bigger social movement for universal healthcare. We must start by sharing our own stories however we're able. One of the most effective ways I've seen stories shared is through the efforts of Little Lobbyists, an advocacy group for children with complex medical needs that was started by Elena Hung and Michelle Morrison, both mothers of children with such needs. They have fought hard to protect healthcare for children like theirs and others, and their passion moves hearts and minds. They have testified on Capitol Hill and met directly with members of Congress, sharing their children's and other children's stories—they've created visibility and garnered media attention, which they amplified through social media.

Activism expert Marshall Ganz writes, "Stories, unlike policy proposals, teach the heart, not just the head. And it is from the heart that we draw our motivation, commitment, and enthusiasm."[17] Imagine the power that can be harnessed from the combined energy of our personal stories about the need for universal coverage. Think about how you feel when a friend shares a story about being wronged. It doesn't matter whether she was sexually harassed, passed over for a promotion at work, or denied healthcare because she couldn't afford the insurance; when injustice happens to our friends, we feel outraged. Now, we need to take our outrage and turn it into political energy. We need to see our friends in the faces of women and men we haven't even met. We need to recognize the ways our troubles are replicated over and over throughout the system. Now, we have a social responsibility to be more than angry; we need to gather together in our anger and turn our collective passion into a forceful social movement.

Our message of reform is a simple one. It fits on a T-shirt: *Healthcare is a human right.* We can succeed if health reform ties to American core values and a simple message that galvanizes a broad coalition. We need to wrap this message in themes of patriotism and love of country. This will inspire. This will move us to action at last.

A CRUCIAL STEP on our path to victory involves bringing more women into the political arena. It turns out that women are just as electable as men;

the problem is that women are less likely to run for office. There are many explanations for this: we as women are less likely to see ourselves as qualified, we have more family responsibilities, we know we will face discrimination in the public spotlight, we may not have access to the same donor networks that men do, and the list goes on. To paraphrase feminist scholar Heidi Hartmann, "Men look in the mirror and see a candidate; women don't."[18] This is starting to change. One of my favorite signs at the San Francisco Women's March in 2018 said, "First we march, then we run!" And it was true! More women ran and won in the 2018 congressional midterm elections than ever before. We need to ensure this trend continues—that means many women who haven't previously considered pursuing political office need to seriously examine their own potential to run. Whatever level of government they choose, be it local, state, or federal—the more women, the better. As Congresswoman Maxine Waters famously said at a women's convention in 2017, "We are reclaiming our time."

Granted, not every woman wants to run for office. But every one of us can identify great candidates, encourage them to run, and then support them by hosting campaign events or serving on campaign committees. Just be sure that the candidates you choose support universal healthcare unequivocally. But also, be practical. People may not agree with you on the details of how to get there, but they can still agree on the direction we should be heading. The policy details can get worked out over time, and compromise is inevitable in the political process. A great candidate is one who helps lead public opinion, rather than just follow it. The candidate also needs to demonstrate the ability to persist when the going gets tough. And, while I strongly believe that more women should step up and lead, and be encouraged to lead, it's worth remembering that some of the greatest champions of expanded healthcare coverage have been men, including President Harry Truman, Senator Edward M. Kennedy, and President Barack Obama.

Once candidates are elected to office, we need to take collective action to keep universal healthcare high on their agenda. Demonstrated public support provides resilience for elected officials who face pressures to *not* support universal healthcare. We can show continued support for our elected officials' focus on universal healthcare and demand accountability through phone calls, attendance at town hall meetings, and regular participation in local protests and marches. And of course, for those who can afford it, financial support is critical. Ultimately, this public pressure, along with the media attention it generates and the conversations and connections it fosters along the way (often behind the scenes), will lead to culture change and a political imperative for universal healthcare. We can shift public opinion enough to overcome more narrow and powerful industry stakeholder interests.

It will require persistence. You never know how much activism is needed until it's done.[19] One of the biggest lessons we learned from the ACA is that a major health reform law needs to inspire support before *and* after it passes. As former White House advisors Jeanne Lambrew and Ellen Montz write, "Even the most technically sound policy will fall short if it does not generate and sustain pressure for continuing expansion and improvement."[20]

PROTECTING THE ACA

"Nobody dies because they don't have access to health care." Former Republican congressman Raúl Labrador's now infamous remark was made during a 2017 town hall meeting while he was pushing to repeal the ACA. Fortunately, the cacophony of "boos" that followed was a proud showing of the understanding, awareness, and energy of the activists in Idaho who spent their time fighting to ensure that people in their state are able to obtain affordable health insurance, even if their elected officials sometimes neglect to do so.

As we work toward universal healthcare, we have to be ever-vigilant and be sure that we protect the coverage gains we've made. It's vital to be informed and stay active. If we don't keep the pressure on, many state and federal officials will become increasingly confident in their abilities to erode the law. They are likely to keep trying, and we can't let "repeal and replace" fatigue prevent us from marching in the streets when they do.

The pressure has worked before. The public outcry in response to attempts to repeal the ACA was tremendous. Again and again, people spilled into the streets wielding clever, caustic, and poignant signs, voicing their opposition, listening to expert speakers, and intermingling with like-minded activists. Ultimately, the strategy worked. Even though Republicans had control over the House, Senate, and presidency, and had made a number of verbal commitments to repeal and replace the ACA, their efforts failed.

STATE-LEVEL ACTION

States can act even when the federal government doesn't. In the absence of full universal healthcare, states can protect the ACA and support Medicaid expansion within their own borders. We can help push them to do this. With on-the-ground pragmatism, we can help state elected officials recognize the economic reality of uninsured citizens and underfunded safety net or rural hospitals.

To protect the ACA, states can pass laws to help keep premiums from getting too high and to ensure more coverage. California did just this in 2019 with its law establishing more generous health insurance subsidies along with an individual mandate. Several other states have taken action, including New Jersey, Rhode Island and Vermont (which have all established individual mandates), as well as Connecticut: anticipating the possibility that federal protections for essential health benefits were to discontinue, the Connecticut legislature passed a bill in 2018 enshrining them in state law and ensuring that men continued to contribute equally to services that women use and everyone benefits from.[21]

State Medicaid expansion policy is also highly responsive to political activism. If the remaining fourteen states were to expand their Medicaid programs, 4.5 million Americans would gain Medicaid coverage, over half of whom would be newly insured. If you live in one of the few remaining holdout states, you have a few routes for effective advocacy.[22]

One is a ballot initiative—only some states allow them, but in those that do, it's a great way to get involved. You can support or join an advocacy group trying to get a veto-proof expansion law passed. (That's right, if a voter-sponsored referendum is passed, it's veto-proof, which means the governor can't undo it.) To get an initiative on the ballot requires signatures, so helping collect them is an important task. Once the initiative is on the ballot, a more traditional campaign will ensue to increase support and help the initiative win at the ballot box.

If you live in a state that doesn't allow ballot initiatives, you can still lobby the state's legislature or get involved with advocacy groups. You can write letters to your elected officials or even meet with them. Resistance to Medicaid expansion is waning the longer the ACA has been in place. State officials are having a difficult time explaining to their constituents why they shouldn't be eligible for this program, which is mostly federally funded. Resisters have capitulated one by one: Alaska, Indiana, Louisiana, Montana, New Hampshire, Pennsylvania, and Virginia initially refused expansion but eventually decided to join in, and they were followed by Maine, Nebraska, Idaho, and Utah via citizen-sponsored ballot initiatives.[23] Citizens in those states were fed up with governing officials who were resisting Medicaid expansion, and they pursued voter-sponsored ballot initiatives to expand the program and largely succeeded.

If you don't live in any of these states, you can still support their efforts by donating to the advocacy organizations that are trying to expand Medicaid in their states. Outside of political involvement, you can take action within your own family or community to increase coverage. Millions of children in this country are eligible for Medicaid or CHIP, yet still don't have it. If you have a child or know a child who is currently uninsured, you can gather knowledge about the requirements for Medicaid and CHIP from your state and/or direct them to a navigator organization to help to get them covered if they are eligible. Similarly, if you know adults who are uninsured or underinsured, you can talk to them about their options for coverage.

ADDRESSING SOCIAL DETERMINANTS OF HEALTH

As I showed in chapter 7, we need to think beyond coverage expansion to other important factors that determine our health—this includes addressing inequality. We have to "recognize the ill effects that American underinvestment in social services and inattention to social capital have had on health."[24] Remember: other countries invest in universal coverage *and* social services. They have also taken steps to reduce inequality through their approach to social and tax policy. They provide more supports to new parents, the unemployed, and the next generation. We have many ways to do that in the US, including through expansion of the earned income tax credit and supports for families, like paid leave and childcare.

We need to address the so-called upstream (societal and structural) issues. Fortunately, some industry leaders and politicians are aware of the limitations of the $3.65 trillion healthcare industry. These forward-looking leaders are redirecting their attention and resources upstream, away from healthcare, where they can have more impact. We're already seeing the health system begin to endorse and/or link to programs that promote healthy living environments, community engagement, housing supports, healthy food, education, and more. We can support them and push them to do more. We've got a long way to go, but we're moving in the right direction. Pursuing universal healthcare and addressing the nonmedical determinants of health are complementary goals.

GET INVOLVED!

As women, we are united. Many of us understand and share the burden of caregiving, and we draw strength from one another and our community. We can and should bridge some of the partisan divide and find pragmatic solutions. We can connect through the humanitarian things we have in common: protecting our children and families, supporting our friends and communities. We can tap into our patriotism and love of America. Together, we can strengthen our social fabric and the quilt of coverage. Women can establish healthcare as a right in the US if we tap into our full potential, collectively and individually.

As I said at the outset, social movements are aspirational. To be successful, they also require other elements, including grassroots organizing, seizing opportunities when they arise, and building incrementally toward long-term goals. Within this framework, there are roles for everyone. All of us can ask candidates, "What's your plan for universal healthcare?" With financial donations, we can be "patrons of political action." The social movements of the 1960s and '70s also had patrons who gave money to mobilize and support collective action.

Whether it's supporting universal healthcare, protecting the ACA, promoting state legislation, or addressing social determinants, the key is to get involved with *something* that will improve our collective health. Find what you believe in most—there are so many possibilities. My passion and expertise unite around pushing for universal coverage, but I recognize that it won't eliminate all health disparities, so I try to work on social determinants as well, through volunteering in the Somerville public schools, donating, and more.

Carving out even a little time will help. Kara Waite's story is an example of how you can be politically active with limited time. Kara is an English teacher at Bunker Hill Community College in Charlestown, Massachusetts, who "made a rule for herself: For every political rant she posts on Facebook, she must pick up the phone and call a legislator." Kara sets a calendar reminder to call party leadership every Monday morning. She said that "first-time callers often fear they will be quizzed or interrogated, but that they generally just need to offer their opinion and basic personal information, like name and city."[25] What's great about this kind of participation is that it makes a difference. As US senator Kirsten Gillibrand explained, "It helps that I get thousands of phone calls every day on an issue because then when I'm giving a speech on the Senate floor, I can talk about the passion of my constituents and I can talk about letters that people have actually written me and share those stories to millions of people. So, you are projecting your voice when you make those calls regardless of who you are calling."[26]

And there's always more that we can do—I've included a "Take Action" resource list on my website, https://rosemarieday.com.

E VEN THOUGH MUCH of the energy around healthcare reform historically has been devoted to making change incrementally and at the community level, we need to advocate for a full solution to affordable health coverage now. We need to build on women's history of activism and push forward even more. If social movements are made up of a series of moments, now is one of those moments.

Let's be inspired and fueled by passion, while also staying laser-focused on practical solutions. We can be idealistic, we can be mad—all of these emotions provide good energy that we need to harness to fuel a social movement. At the same time, we need to be practical. Relentlessly so. We need to find that calm spot in the storm and persist.

So if you believe in healthcare as a right, then you need to look beyond the ACA's shortcomings, help to find and support universal healthcare solutions, and continue to push forward to affordable universal coverage. We need to keep our eyes on the horizon and prepare for the next opportunity. We need to create a wave of support for affordable universal coverage. In fact, we should make it a tsunami!

We've made a good start—women triumphed in the 2018 congressional midterm elections and healthcare was a major issue for voters. The momentum is building. I'm encouraged to see a record number of women running for president in 2020. Seeing a woman running for higher office is beginning to feel more normal and it's great to have so many choices.

But having more women in office is not enough. It all comes back to you. Make affordable universal healthcare your priority issue and encourage others to do the same. Together, we can be inspired by women's history of activism and build a national movement for universal healthcare.

That's never been clearer to me than when the first Women's March on Washington was drawing to a close. Late that afternoon, we walked past an area where people were pausing to dispose of their signs, and as a small group gathered, an impromptu chorus began singing anthems of the civil rights movement, songs like "We Shall Overcome" and "Amazing Grace." Remarkably, a guitarist joined us, too, and in that moment, as I raised my voice, I was struck by the connection I felt to the activists who have come before me. Like them, I recognize injustice—this time it's in our healthcare system. And like them, I have witnessed the power of peaceful protest and collective action. I understand that at times, progress may seem slower and more incremental than I'd like. But I also know that together, we can create positive change as we work toward recognition of healthcare as a right for all Americans.

As Rosa Parks said, "We must not be afraid to take the first step." I sincerely hope that you will join me as a healthcare activist, and that I've inspired you to take the first step, and then, the next.

ON A PERSONAL NOTE

A surplus of effort could overcome a deficit of confidence.

—SONIA SOTOMAYOR,
first Latina Supreme Court Justice[1]

A S I CONCLUDE THIS BOOK, I want to come full circle and bring things back to a personal level. My healthcare journey became acutely personal when health issues hit my family and me hard in 2017. I told myself that if I survived my cancer and got through that year, I would do something to protect other people's health coverage, so that they could have the financial peace of mind that I was lucky to have. It's hard enough to be sick and manage your treatments without having to worry about how you are going to pay for it. Once I could manage it, I started becoming more visibly political by participating in marches and other activities. Writing this book has been my biggest step so far. I did it because people were asking me during and after the marches, "What more can I do?" I realized I had a lot of knowledge and passion to share, and so I began.

At this point you may be wondering, *Am I really an activist?* Most of us aren't used to thinking about ourselves in those terms, and at first the idea might seem a bit daunting. That's completely understandable. During the Women's March, I spoke with many women who had never participated in public protests before. Others I know didn't march but contributed with social media posts amplifying the message. What can unite us, and bring us to activism, is our emotional energy and our passion for the cause.

New forms of activism can stretch you beyond your comfort zone. Even though I had participated in several marches, I found that I was a bit nervous about joining a movement called #StandOnEveryCorner. It was created to raise awareness about injustice. As much as I know and care about health reform, I hadn't taken such a visible stand as I did when I put myself out there, at a busy intersection in Somerville, holding a sign that read "Believe Women." This small, local protest was so public, and yet so personal. It felt different from participating in larger events, where there is a measure of anonymity. But by accepting the challenge and sticking with it, I've met new friends, expanded my worldview, and learned from others with different styles and approaches.

As I've learned more about activism, I've discovered that one of the biggest misconceptions is that activism is "binary"—you've either devoted your life to a cause or you haven't. But there are many ways to get involved, and you must find whatever works best for you. As *The Everygirl* blogger Daryl Lindsey states so well, "Getting more involved doesn't have to take over your life, and it doesn't have to be the primary facet of your identity. You can support and promote meaningful causes and, yes, change the world, while still being a 'normal' person living a 'normal' life."[2]

As mentioned, to help you determine your comfort level with healthcare activism, I developed a Personal Activism Assessment (see my website, https://rosemarieday.com). Based on your answers, your activism profile will fall into one of these four categories:

- *Awareness.* At this level, you are informally affiliated with healthcare causes beyond your own personal experiences. You are beginning to understand the systemic issues around healthcare coverage and the need for activism. You are focused on gaining knowledge and are comfortable reading, listening to podcasts, and attending talks about the cause.

- *Sharing.* You are still informally affiliated with healthcare causes but are more knowledgeable and have developed some social engagement around them. You may be vocal with people who disagree with you, even if they are beyond your immediate circles of friends and colleagues. You're increasingly comfortable communicating with others in person or online about your ideas or stories related to the cause.

- *Participation.* At this level, you are more formally affiliated with the cause, have more social engagement, and are focusing on direct participation. You show your support by making donations, volunteering, or signing petitions. You may be willing to participate in visible political activism to support healthcare as a human right. You might join an organization dedicated to the cause, attend a town hall meeting, or participate in a protest.

- *Leadership.* You are formally affiliated with the movement for health-care as a right, have a high level of social engagement, and are focused on leadership opportunities. You are very proactive and are willing to organize groups of people to participate in the cause. Your activities span a wide range, from organizing an event, to leading an organization or a campaign dedicated to the cause, to running for office.

Within each of these categories are several dimensions, including your level of time commitment (five minutes versus five hours versus five years) and your degree of exposure (behind-the-scenes roles versus front-line op-portunities). Wherever you land, you need to challenge yourself to move out of your comfort zone to engage even more over time and possibly with higher exposure.

I was challenged to move out of my comfort zone once again (this time in the category of sharing) when my surgeon asked me to speak about my breast cancer diagnosis and treatment at a fundraiser for the center where I was treated. Even though I'm used to public speaking in my professional life, it hasn't been easy for me to tell that personal story, and my immediate reaction was to decline. But I didn't want to disappoint her. So, I said "yes," and then had to work through multiple drafts of my talk and practice in front of my family before I was comfortable taking the stage. And I was glad I did—I got to witness firsthand the power that comes from sharing your personal story.

My mother falls into the category of "sharing" as well, and I used to think of her as an "armchair activist." But she has proven that you're never too old to move out of your comfort zone and become a more public activist! Always knowledgeable about political issues, and very vocal about them around our kitchen table, my mother was most comfortable volunteering in our com-munity, through PTA, Girl Scouts, and the March of Dimes. She took some political action in a local, nonpartisan way, by supporting school committee and city council candidates, as well as the League of Women Voters. But un-til the 2017 Women's March, she had never participated in a public protest. Now, my eighty-three-year-old mother and her friend, also eighty-three, enjoy wearing their pink pussy hats and "nasty women" T-shirts when they go on their exercise walks. They want people to know where they stand on the issues. Many people have asked to take their photo—and they are always more than happy to oblige.

These examples bring up another important point: as you think about ways to get involved, be sure to prioritize in-person options. While doing something online can be easy, since it's always available, online participation won't meet some of your emotional needs. There is tremendous value in connecting with people in person. You will be energized by the connections, and you build your social supports. As Gloria Steinem says, "People in the same room understand and empathize with each other in a way that isn't possible on the page or screen."[3]

Getting involved lifts your spirits, as my childhood friend who worked on expanding Medicaid in Idaho found. She told me that once she "got off the sidelines," she felt less anger and engaged in fewer rants. She said, "Even if we lose, I'm working with great people!" (They won.)

Inviting a friend to join you is an easy way to move into the category of "Participation" or even "Leadership." Rather than thinking of this as an "ask," reframe your approach and think about how you are giving people the opportunity to help. I did this in 2016 when I invited one of my best friends to join me in canvassing in New Hampshire for Hillary Clinton. My friend hadn't gone door to door since she was a Girl Scout in the 1980s and was a little nervous about doing it. But she cared deeply about the election and wanted to be more involved. I gave her that opportunity. The MomsRising folks think of this as "opening doors for people to feel their power."[4] It's an act of generosity to find ways to bring people together and engage them in thinking big. You are helping them to grow and find new sources of support, just as you are for yourself.

To sustain the movement, we must sustain ourselves. After all, many women are already spread too thin with work and family responsibilities. I know how difficult it can be to find the energy to do one more thing. Recognizing that activism doesn't have to take over your life is key. So, start by focusing on what can be accomplished with small bits of time. You can sign up for "action alerts," donate, or share something on social media from your smartphone while you are standing in line at the grocery store or waiting for your take-out order to be ready.

To keep from feeling overwhelmed, set one or two goals and focus on them. Make the goals specific, such as "sign up to volunteer this month," rather than "get more active." Post the goals in a prominent place and do something regularly, so that civic engagement becomes a habit or part of your routine. And be sure to reward yourself—it's likely that advocating for issues you care about will be rewarding on its own, but you should still take a moment and treat yourself to something, especially when you reach an important goal.

As Rosa Parks said, "We must not be afraid to take the first step." I find it helpful to think about the steps like this:

1. *Imagine.* Dare to dream of a better world—dwell in that possibility, and then go for it.
2. *Participate.* Democracy is not a spectator sport—you must participate. And women cannot wait for the level playing field—we need to get out there *now.*
3. *Enjoy.* You will benefit from your involvement, so don't hold back. It's worth it. Working toward positive change is empowering.
4. *Persist.* Be relentless. Change doesn't happen overnight. Creating it can be a marathon, so find ways to keep your energy up.

Now is the time. Join me!

TO COMPLETE YOUR PERSONAL ACTIVISM ASSESSMENT
AND FIND MORE WAYS TO GET INVOLVED,
PLEASE GO TO MY WEBSITE:

HTTPS://ROSEMARIEDAY.COM

GLOSSARY

NOTE: Many of these definitions were obtained from HealthCare.gov. For more extensive descriptions and information about key programs, such as Medicare and Medicaid, please see my website: https://RosemarieDay.com.

ACTUARIAL VALUE. The percentage of total average costs for covered benefits that a plan will cover. Metal ratings on the individual market (bronze, silver, gold, etc.) refer to a plan's actuarial value.

ADVANCE PREMIUM TAX CREDIT (APTC). A tax credit you can take in advance to lower your monthly health insurance payment (or "premium"). APTCs are available only for plans sold on the Health Insurance Marketplace.

CENTER OF EXCELLENCE (COE). A program within a healthcare institution that is assembled to supply an exceptionally high concentration of expertise and related resources centered on a particular area of medicine.[1]

CHILDREN'S HEALTH INSURANCE PROGRAM (CHIP). An insurance program that provides low-cost health coverage to children in families that earn too much money to qualify for Medicaid but not enough to buy private insurance. In some states, CHIP covers pregnant women.

COINSURANCE. The percentage of costs of a covered healthcare service you pay (20 percent, for example) after you've paid your deductible.

CONSOLIDATED OMNIBUS BUDGET RECONCILIATION ACT (COBRA). A federal law that may allow you to temporarily keep health coverage after your employment ends or you lose coverage as a dependent of the covered employee or have another qualifying event. If you elect COBRA coverage, you pay 100 percent of the premiums, including the share the employer used to pay, plus a small administrative fee.

CO-PAYMENT. A fixed amount ($20, for example) you pay for a covered healthcare service after you've paid your deductible.

DEDUCTIBLE. The amount you pay for covered healthcare services before your insurance plan starts to pay.

EXCHANGE. An online service available in every state that helps individuals, families, and small businesses shop for and enroll in health insurance. Also known as Health Insurance Marketplace.

FEDERAL POVERTY LEVEL (FPL). A measure of income set every year by the Department of Health and Human Services (HHS). Federal poverty levels are used to determine your eligibility for certain programs and benefits, including savings on Marketplace health insurance, and Medicaid and CHIP coverage.

HEALTH INSURANCE MARKETPLACE. Another term for Exchange, an online service available in every state that helps individuals, families, and small businesses shop for and enroll in health insurance.

HEALTH SAVINGS ACCOUNT (HSA). A type of savings account that lets you set aside money on a pretax basis to pay for qualified medical expenses.

HIGH-DEDUCTIBLE HEALTH PLAN (HDHP). For 2020, the IRS defines a high-deductible health plan as any plan with a deductible of at least $1,400 for an individual or $2,800 for a family.

INPATIENT. Medical care that requires a patient to stay overnight in a hospital or other health facility.

LONG-TERM CARE. Services that include medical and nonmedical care provided to people who are unable to perform basic activities of daily living such as dressing or bathing.

MEDICAID. An insurance program that provides free or low-cost health coverage to low-income people, including families and children, pregnant women, the elderly, and people with disabilities.

MEDICARE. A federal health insurance program for people sixty-five and older and certain younger people with disabilities. It also covers people with End-Stage Renal Disease (permanent kidney failure requiring dialysis or a transplant, sometimes called ESRD).

MEDICARE ADVANTAGE. Also known as Medicare Part C. A type of Medicare health plan offered by a private company that contracts with Medicare to provide Part A and Part B benefits.

MEDICARE PART A. A component of Medicare to which eligible Americans are automatically enrolled and that pays for hospital bills.

MEDICARE PART B. A component of Medicare for which eligible Americans must pay a small premium to enroll and that pays for outpatient care, physician services, and tests.

MEDICARE PART D. A program that helps pay for prescription drugs for people with Medicare who join a plan that includes Medicare prescription drug coverage.

NONGROUP. Individual health insurance that is bought by and covers an individual person or a family instead of having been purchased by a group (such as a company or a union) or provided as a benefit by the government.

OUT-OF-POCKET MAXIMUM. The most you have to pay for covered services in a plan year. After you spend this amount on deductibles, co-payments, and co-insurance, your health plan pays 100 percent of the costs of covered benefits.

OUTPATIENT. Medical care that does not require a patient to stay overnight. Also referred to as ambulatory care.

PATIENT PROTECTION AND AFFORDABLE CARE ACT. The comprehensive healthcare reform law enacted in March 2010 (sometimes known as ACA, PPACA, or "Obamacare").

PREEXISTING CONDITION. A health problem, like asthma, diabetes, or cancer, you had before the date that new health coverage starts. In the practical sense, this term refers to the health conditions that, if you had them, would cause an insurance company to increase your premiums or refuse to sell you a plan before the ACA outlawed this practice.

PREMIUM. The amount you pay for your health insurance every month.

PRIMARY CARE. Health services that cover a range of prevention, wellness, and treatment for common illnesses.

READMISSION. An incident in which a patient unexpectedly returns to the hospital soon after being discharged.

RESCISSION. The retroactive cancellation of a health insurance policy. Under the Affordable Care Act, rescission is illegal except in cases of fraud or intentional misrepresentation of material fact as prohibited by the terms of the plan or coverage.

RISK ADJUSTMENT. A statistical process that takes into account the underlying health status and health spending of the enrollees in an insurance plan when looking at their healthcare outcomes or healthcare costs.

RISK POOL. A group of people, covered by health insurance, who are grouped together to calculate premiums so that those with high cost and those with low cost balance one another out.

SELF-INSURED. A type of plan usually present in larger companies where the employer itself collects premiums from enrollees and takes on the responsibility of paying employees' and dependents' medical claims. These employers can contract for insurance services such as enrollment, claims processing, and provider networks with a third party administrator, or they can be self-administered.

SPECIALIST. A physician specialist focuses on a specific area of medicine or a group of patients to diagnose, manage, prevent, or treat certain types of symptoms and conditions.

UNCOMPENSATED CARE. Healthcare or services provided by hospitals or healthcare providers that don't get reimbursed. Often uncompensated care arises when people don't have insurance and cannot afford to pay the cost of care.

UNDERINSURED. People with high deductibles and out-of-pocket costs relative to their incomes. Low-income families are underinsured if they spend more than 5 percent of their incomes on these expenses. High-income families are underinsured if they spend more than 10 percent of their incomes on these expenses.[2]

VALUE-BASED CARE. An increasingly common reimbursement arrangement in which healthcare providers are compensated for providing high-quality care at low cost rather than for each specific service rendered.

ACKNOWLEDGMENTS

As with any big project in life, it truly "takes a village" to get it done. I am deeply grateful to all of the people who believe in this cause and have helped me to make this book a reality.

First, to my team at Day Health Strategies: you are truly an incredible group of people. You combine so many great qualities, including high levels of intelligence and problem-solving talent, with dedication to making the world a better place. You have provided tremendous support throughout this project. Thank you especially to Niko Lehman-White, who did so much research and development of the book's foundational pieces, and to Emily Eibl, for her research, support, and feminist perspective. And thank you to Sarah Bliss Matousek, Lisette Roman, and Ross Weiler for your insights and for stepping up to lead when I really had to buckle down and write! Thank you also to our firm's advisors, who have helped us to see the path forward for many years, especially Laura Downing and Russ Moran.

Next, I owe a huge thank-you to Kathryn Siranosian, who collaborated with me throughout the entire project: you taught me a lot about writing and always saw the forest through the trees. Thank you for cheering me on and sharing my feminist spirit and passion for the cause!

I also want to thank everyone who reviewed portions (or more!) of this book and provided invaluable advice, including Linda Blumberg, John Mc-Donough, and Roosa Tikkanen. Thank you also to those who contributed input and answered my questions, including Larry Levitt, Jane Mansbridge, and Kristin Rowe-Finkbeiner. The book is much better for it.

My team at Beacon Press has been incredible, especially in making this book more "feminist-forward." Thank you especially to Helene Atwan and Haley Lynch for believing in a first-time author!

In addition, I am grateful for all of my professional role models, mentors, and sponsors: I wouldn't be where I am today without your support and inspiration. A special thank-you goes to my first boss at the YWCA, Kay Philips, and to the many other bosses who gave me opportunities along the way, including Becky Morgan, Claire McIntire, Wendy Warring, David Ellwood, Jon Kingsdale, and Charlie Baker.

To my incredible women friends, whose support through *all* of life's challenges has been steadfast and immense, including the Moms Group (Wendy Gulley, Sheridan Kahmann, Laura Lever, and Meg O'Leary—we are Momstrong!) and my other "sisters" (Kathy Parker Boudett, Allison Chang, Diane Gosney, and Wanda McClain). I love you all!

Thank you also to the women who participated in my activism workshop to help make this book more empowering, including Kathy Boudett, Tiziana Dearing, Deb Gordon, Wanda McClain, Kathy Siranosian, and Linda Viens. You inspire me!

I also want to thank my amazing care team from the Hoffman Breast Center at Mt. Auburn Hospital: Dr. Susan Pories, Dr. Lisa Weissmann, and Dr. Terri Silver. You are an incredible team—so smart, strong, caring, and collaborative. My life was in your hands, and this book is one of many ways I hope to thank you.

And finally, I owe a huge debt of gratitude to my wonderful family: my husband, Steve Churchill, who has been such a loving and steady presence in my life for more than thirty years, providing liberal doses of humor and unwavering support for every one of my challenging endeavors; and to my three children, Kate, Andrew, and Ellie, who bring me great joy and who manage to love their "nontraditional" mom. And to my parents, who gave me so much. I love you all, more than I can say.

NOTES

PREFACE

1. James A. Morone and David Blumenthal, "The Arc of History Bends toward Coverage: Health Policy at a Crossroads," *Health Affairs* 37, no. 3 (2018): 351–57, doi:10.1377/hlthaff .2017.1312.

CHAPTER 1: WHY COVERAGE MATTERS

1. Maxwell Ubah, *The HOW of Leadership: Inspire People to Achieve Extraordinary Results* (New York: Business Expert Press, 2018).

2. Liz Hamel et al., "Survey of Non-Group Health Insurance Enrollees, Wave 3," Henry J. Kaiser Family Foundation, July 13, 2016, https://www.kff.org/health-reform/poll-finding /survey-of-non-group-health-insurance-enrollees-wave-3.

3. "Fact Sheet: General Facts on Women and Job Based Health," US Department of Labor, Employee Benefits Security Administration, https://www.dol.gov/sites/dolgov/files/EBSA /about-ebsa/our-activities/resource-center/fact-sheets/women-and-job-based-health.pdf.

4. Carolyn Buck Luce, *Reimagining Healthcare: Through a Gender Lens* (Los Angeles: Rare Bird Books, 2016), 7.

5. Z. Byron Wolf, "Is There Something Wrong with This White House Photo?," CNN, March 24, 2017, https://www.cnn.com/2017/03/23/politics/mike-pence-patty-murray-photo /index.html.

6. "The 1965 Medicare Amendment to the Social Security Act," LBJ Presidential Library, August 27, 2012, http://www.lbjlibrary.org/press/the-1965-medicare-amendment-to-the-social -security-act.

7. David Himmelstein et al., "Medical Bankruptcy—Q&A," Physicians for a National Health Program, http://www.pnhp.org/sites/default/files/docs/Medical-Bankruptcy-Q-and -A.pdf.

8. Steffie Woolhandler and David Himmelstein, "The Relationship of Health Insurance and Mortality: Is Lack of Insurance Deadly?," *Annals of Internal Medicine* 167, no. 6 (2017): 424, doi:10.7326/m17-1403.

9. "Universal Declaration of Human Rights," United Nations, http://www.un.org/en /universal-declaration-human-rights.

10. John Rawls, *Justice as Fairness: A Restatement* (1985; New York: Irvington, 2001), 174.

11. For a more in-depth discussion on this topic, please read Gunnar Almgren's wonderful book, *Health Care as a Right of Citizenship: The Continuing Evolution of Reform* (New York: Columbia University Press, 2017).

12. Alicia Oken, "Weekly Wrap Up: 'No One Should Go Broke Just Because They Get Sick,'" National Archives and Records Administration, September 27, 2013, https://obama whitehouse.archives.gov/blog/2013/09/27/weekly-wrap-no-one-should-go-broke-just-because -they-get-sick.

13. Ricardo Alonso-Zaldivar and Laurie Kellman, "NORC Poll: Shift to Political Left Seen on Health Care," Associated Press-NORC Center for Public Affairs Research, July 20, 2017, http://www.apnorc.org/news-media/Pages/AP-NORC-Poll-Shift-to-political-left-seen -on-health-care.aspx.

14. Eighty-six percent of women versus 75 percent of men believe it should be illegal to deny coverage to people with preexisting conditions. "National Tracking Poll #180919," Morning Consult, September 9, 2018, https://morningconsult.com/wp-content/uploads/2018/09 /180919_crosstabs_POLITICO_v1_DK.pdf.

15. "Repealing the Individual Health Insurance Mandate: An Updated Estimate," Congressional Budget Office, November 2017, https://www.cbo.gov/system/files/115th-congress -2017-2018/reports/53300-individualmandate.pdf.

CHAPTER 2: HOW WE GOT HERE AND WHERE WE STAND

1. "Transcript of Pelosi, Hoyer, Clyburn Press Conference Highlighting Benefits of Affordable Care Act," last modified March 23, 2012, https://www.speaker.gov/newsroom /transcript-pelosi-hoyer-clyburn-press-conference-highlighting-benefits-affordable -care-act.

2. For a good summary, see Morone and Blumenthal, "The Arc of History Bends toward Coverage: 351–57, doi:10.1377/hlthaff.2017.1312. For a more in-depth summary, see chapter 5 of Ezekiel Emanuel, *Reinventing American Health Care: How the Affordable Care Act Will Improve Our Terribly Complex, Blatantly Unjust, Outrageously Expensive, Grossly Inefficient, Error Prone System* (New York: PublicAffairs, 2014).

3. Gunnar Almgren, *Health Care Politics, Policy, and Services: A Social Justice Analysis* (New York: Springer, 2018), 49.

4. Emanuel, *Reinventing American Health Care*, 133.

5. Harry Truman, *Memoirs*, vol. 1: *Years of Trial and Hope, 1946–1952* (New York: Doubleday, 1955), 19.

6. Emanuel, *Reinventing American Health Care*, 30.

7. Emanuel, *Reinventing American Health Care*, 31.

8. This began during World War II as an IRS decision and was put into law in the 1950s during President Eisenhower's term.

9. Julie Rovner, "The Huge (and Rarely Discussed) Health Insurance Tax Break," NPR, December 4, 2012, https://www.npr.org/sections/health-shots/2012/12/04/166434247/the -huge-and-rarely-discussed-health-insurance-tax-break.

10. Morone and Blumenthal, "The Arc of History."

11. This was the infamous "Harry and Louise" ad campaign, a series of fourteen commercials with "devastating impact." Emanuel, *Reinventing*, 151.

12. John McDonough, *Inside National Health Reform* (London: University of California Press, 2011), 24.

13. Ryan Grim, "Why Getting Beaten by Your Husband Is a Pre-Existing Condition," *Huffington Post*, November 14, 2009, https://www.huffingtonpost.com/2009/09/14/when-getting-beaten-by-yo_n_286029.html.

14. "Hearing Before the Subcommittee on Oversight and Investigations of the Committee on Energy and Commerce," June 16, 2009, https://www.gpo.gov/fdsys/pkg/CHRG -111hhrg73743/html/CHRG-111hhrg73743.htm.

15. "Hearing Before the Subcommittee on Oversight and Investigations of the Committee on Energy and Commerce," June 16, 2009, https://www.gpo.gov/fdsys/pkg/CHRG -111hhrg73743/html/CHRG-111hhrg73743.htm.

16. For a wonderful description of this process, see McDonough, *Inside National Health Reform*.

17. Most notably, Senator Max Baucus (Democrat from Montana) spent months courting moderate Republicans. It was to no avail, however—Senator Olympia Snowe (Republican

from Maine) was the last holdout, and eventually she made the political calculation to side with the Republicans and oppose the ACA.

18. Cecile Richards and Lauren Peterson, *Make Trouble: Standing Up, Speaking Out, and Finding the Courage to Lead* (New York: Gallery Books, 2019), 194.

19. "Today, We Have the Opportunity to Complete the Great Unfinished Business of Our Society and Pass Health Insurance Reform for All Americans," Nancy Pelosi, Speaker of the House, March 21, 2010, https://www.speaker.gov/newsroom/pelosi-todayopportunity -complete-great-unfinished-business-society-pass-health-insurance-reform-americans.

20. "Health Care Bill Signing Ceremony," C-SPAN, March 23, 2010, https://www.c-span .org/video/?292681-1/health-care-bill-signing-ceremony.

21. Jason Mattera, "Gingrich Calls Obamacare 'Centralized Healthcare Dictatorship,'" Human Events, January 19, 2011, http://humanevents.com/2011/01/19/gingrich-calls-obamacare -centralized-healthcare-dictatorship.

22. Marvin Olasky, "Don't Forget Obamacare," World Magazine, October 23, 2010, https://world.wng.org/2010/10/dont_forget_obamacare.

23. Edwin Meese III and Robert Alt, "Kasich Is Wrong about Reagan," *National Review*, October 21, 2013, https://www.nationalreview.com/2013/10/kasich-wrong-about-reagan -edwin-meese-iii-robert-alt.

24. Kevin Liptak, "Trump: 'Nobody Knew Health Care Could Be So Complicated,'" CNN, February 28, 2017, https://www.cnn.com/2017/02/27/politics/trump-health-care -complicated/index.html.

25. "American Health Care Act," Congressional Budget Office, last modified March 13, 2017, https://www.cbo.gov/publication/52486; "H.R. 1628, Obamacare Repeal Reconciliation Act of 2017," Congressional Budget Office, last modified July 19, 2017, https://www.cbo.gov /publication/52939.

26. "Americans' Views on Replacing the ACA," AP NORC, http://apnorc.org/projects /Pages/Americans-Views-on-Replacing-the-ACA.aspx.

27. Jonathan Martin and Alexander Burns, "Governors from Both Parties Denounce Senate Obamacare Repeal Bill," *New York Times*, July 14, 2017, https://www.nytimes.com/2017/07 /14/us/politics/governors-oppose-senate-affordable-care-act-repeal.html; Benjamin Swasey, "Baker And 9 Other Governors Ask Senators to Reject Graham-Cassidy Health Bill," *CommonHealth*, WBUR, September 19, 2017, https://www.wbur.org/commonhealth/2017/09/19 /baker-letter-graham-cassidy.

28. Cam Donaldson and Karen Gerard, "Market Failure in Health Care," in *Economics of Health Care Financing: The Visible Hand* (London: Palgrave, 1993).

29. Bradley Sawyer and Daniel McDermott, "How Does the Quality of the U.S. Healthcare System Compare to Other Countries?" Peterson-Kaiser Health System Tracker, last updated March 28, 2019, https://www.healthsystemtracker.org/chart-collection/quality-u-s -healthcare-system-compare-countries/#item-30-day-mortality-heart-attacks-ischemic -stroke-lower-u-s-comparable-countries.

CHAPTER 3: WHY WOMEN CAN BE THE DRIVERS OF UNIVERSAL HEALTHCARE

1. Sheryl Sandberg, *Lean In for Graduates* (New York: Alfred A. Knopf, 2014), 80.

2. Richards and Peterson, *Make Trouble*, 253.

3. Janie Velencia, "The 2018 Gender Gap Was Huge," *FiveThirtyEight*, November 9, 2018, https://fivethirtyeight.com/features/the-2018-gender-gap-was-huge.

4. "Women in the U.S. Congress 2019," *Center for American Women in Politics*, January 23, 2019, http://www.cawp.rutgers.edu/women-us-congress-2019; Kristin Rowe-Finkbeiner, *Keep Marching: How Every Woman Can Take Action and Change Our World* (New York: Hachette, 2018), 42.

5. Deborah Rhode, *What Women Want: An Agenda for the Women's Movement* (Oxford, UK: Oxford University Press, 2014), 157.

6. Robert Fulghum Quotes, Successories, last updated 2019, https://www.successories.com/iquote/author/13014/robert-fulghum-quotes/1.

7. Title IX was instrumental in opening up educational opportunities for women. Known for covering sports, Title IX granted equal participation in any education program. It also prohibited sex discrimination in education programs, and is often relevant in addressing sexual harassment and violence complaints in schools.

8. Beatrix Hoffman, "Health Care Reform and Social Movements in the United States," *American Journal of Public Health* (January 2003): 75–85, doi:10.2105/ajph.93.1.75.

9. Barbara Seaman, "Health Activism, American Feminist," *Jewish Women: A Comprehensive Historical Encyclopedia*, March 20, 2009, https://jwa.org/encyclopedia/article/health-activism-american-feminist.

10. Rebecca Traister, *Good and Mad: How Women's Anger Is Reshaping America* (New York: Simon & Schuster, 2018), 25.

11. Hoffman, "Health Care Reform and Social Movements in the United States," 75–85.

12. Traister, *Good and Mad*, 42.

13. Hoffman, "Health Care Reform and Social Movements in the United States," 75–85.

14. "Rich Women Begin a War on Cancer," *New York Times*, April 23, 1913; see, also, http://www.mnwelldir.org/docs/history/images/rich women war on cancer 1913.pdf.

15. Susan Smith, *Sick and Tired of Being Sick and Tired: Black Women's Health Activism in America, 1890-1950* (Philadelphia: University of Pennsylvania Press, 1995).

16. Smith, *Sick and Tired of Being Sick and Tired*, 1.

17. Evelynn Hammonds, review of Susan L. Smith, *Sick and Tired of Being Sick and Tired: Black Women's Health Activism in America, 1890-1950, Bulletin of the History of Medicine* 72, no. 1 (Spring 1998): 158–59, http://www.jstor.org/stable/44451525.

18. Smith, *Sick and Tired of Being Sick and Tired*, 8.

19. Angela Castellanos, "Federal Government and African American Communities Identifying and Defining African American Health Disparities through Intervention: The National Negro Health Week Movement and Office of Negro Health Work from 1915–1951," doctoral diss., 2015, Harvard University Medical School, https://dash.harvard.edu/handle/1/17295895.

20. Jennifer Nelson, "'Hold Your Head Up and Stick Out Your Chin': Community Health and Women's Health in Mound Bayou, Mississippi," *NWSA Journal* 17, no. 1 (2005): 99-118, doi:10.2979/nws.2005.17.1.99, 105.

21. Nelson, "'Hold Your Head Up,'" 20–22.

22. Nelson, "'Hold Your Head Up.'"

23. Nelson, "'Hold Your Head Up.'"

24. Smith, *Sick and Tired of Being Sick and Tired*, 14.

25. Soumya Karlamangla, "Male Doctors Are Disappearing from Gynecology. Not Everybody Is Thrilled About It," *Los Angeles Times*, March 7, 2018, https://www.latimes.com/health/la-me-male-gynos-20180307-htmlstory.html.

26. Anne Donchin, "Feminist Bioethics," Stanford Encyclopedia of Philosophy, July 19, 2004, https://stanford.library.sydney.edu.au/archives/fall2008/entries/feminist-bioethics.

27. Nick Davies, "Library of Congress Picks Its 88 Most Influential Books," Melville House Books, June 27, 2012, https://www.mhpbooks.com/library-of-congress-picks-its-88-most-influential-books.

28. Donchin, "Feminist Bioethics."

29. Seaman, "Health Activism, American Feminist."

30. Nelson, "'Hold Your Head Up.'"

31. Sekai Turner, "The National Black Women's Health Project, 1983–1995: A Movement of Inclusive Health Care for Girls and Women," PhD diss., Cornell University, 2010, https://ecommons.cornell.edu.

32. Hoffman, "Health Care Reform and Social Movements in the United States," 75–85.

33. Cecile Richards, "The Affordable Care Act Benefits Women," *Huffington Post*, December 7, 2017, https://www.huffpost.com/entry/the-affordable-care-act-b_b_736927.

34. "U.S. Women's Movements and Health Care Reform," US National Library of Medicine, December 17, 2015, https://circulatingnow.nlm.nih.gov/2015/12/17/u-s-womens-movements-and-health-care-reform-2.

35. Katty Kay and Claire Shipman, "The Confidence Gap," *Atlantic*, May 2014, https://www.theatlantic.com/magazine/archive/2014/05/the-confidence-gap/359815.

36. Traister, *Good and Mad*, xxiv.

37. Traister, *Good and Mad*, 153.

38. Traister, *Good and Mad*, xxxi.

39. Traister, *Good and Mad*, 41.

40. Traister, *Good and Mad*, xxxi.

41. Traister, *Good and Mad*, xx.

CHAPTER 4: EMPLOYER-SPONSORED INSURANCE WON'T SAVE US

1. Thomas L. Friedman, *Thank You for Being Late: An Optimist's Guide to Thriving in the Age of Accelerations* (New York: Farrar, Straus and Giroux, 2015), 239.

2. Joe Alper, *Health Insurance and Insights from Health Literacy: Helping Consumers Understand: Proceedings of a Workshop* (Washington, DC: National Academies Press, 2017); Cathryn Donaldson, "Majority of Americans Satisfied with Their Employer's Health Plan, New Survey Shows," AHIP, February 6, 2018, https://www.ahip.org/majority-of-americans-satisfied-with-their-employers-health-plan-new-survey-shows.

3. *Women in the Labor Force: A Databook*, US Bureau of Labor Statistics, 2017, https://www.bls.gov/opub/reports/womens-databook/2017/home.htm.

4. Of women in the workforce, 90 percent are eligible for employer-sponsored insurance coverage through their own jobs, versus. 93.4 percent of men. Of that, 74.4 percent of women take up the coverage, versus 80.6 percent of men. Bowen Garrett, Len M. Nicholas, and Emily K. Greenman, *Workers Without Health Insurance: Who Are They and How Can Policy Reach Them?* (Battle Creek, MI: Urban Institute, 2019), https://www.urban.org/sites/default/files/publication/61271/310244-Workers-Without-Health-Insurance.PDF. Data was updated for the author by Bowen Garrett in May, 2019, using Tabulations of Integrated Public Use Microdata Series, Current Population Survey Data (IPUMS-CPS), University of Minnesota, www.ipums.org.

5. Natalie Shure, "The Feminist Case for Single Payer," *Jacobin*, December 8, 2017, https://jacobinmag.com/2017/12/single-payer-feminism-medicare-for-all-health-women.

6. Shure, "The Feminist Case for Single Payer."

7. Beth Umland, "Behind in Pay Behind in Benefits," Mercer, October 17, 2014, https://www.mercer.us/our-thinking/healthcare/behind-in-pay-behind-in-benefits.html.

8. Megan Dunn, "Who Chooses Part-Time Work and Why?" US Bureau of Labor Statistics, March 2018, https://www.bls.gov/opub/mlr/2018/article/pdf/who-chooses-part-time-work-and-why.pdf.

9. Shure, "The Feminist Case for Single Payer."

10. "Labor Force Statistics from the Current Population Survey," US Bureau of Labor Statistics, last modified January 18, 2019, https://www.bls.gov/cps/cpsaat08.htm.

11. William Carroll and Edward Miller, "Differences in Health Insurance Coverage between Part-Time and Full-Time Private-Sector Workers, 2005 and 2015," *Agency for Healthcare Research and Quality*, April 2018, https://meps.ahrq.gov/data_files/publications/st511/stat511.shtml.

12. Shure, "The Feminist Case for Single Payer."

13. Shure, "The Feminist Case for Single Payer."

14. Shure, "The Feminist Case for Single Payer."

15. Alison Kodjak, "Trump Guts Requirement that Employer Health Plans Pay for Birth Control," *NPR*, October 6, 2017, https://www.npr.org/sections/health-shots/2017/10/06/555970210/trump-ends-requirement-that-employer-health-plans-pay-for-birth-control.

16. Richard Wolf, "Second Federal Judge Blocks Trump Contraception Rule," *USA To-day*, December 21, 2017, https://www.usatoday.com/story/news/politics/2017/12/21/second-federal-judge-blocks-trump-contraception-rule/974820001.

17. Nancy Tomes, *Remaking the American Patient: How Madison Avenue and Modern Medicine Turned Patients into Consumers* (Chapel Hill: University of North Carolina Press, 2016), 141.

18. The take-up rate of employer-sponsored insurance has declined from 82 percent to 76 percent during the past decade. "Employer Health Benefits," Kaiser Family Foundation, 2018, http://files.kff.org/attachment/Report-Employer-Health-Benefits-Annual-Survey-2018.

19. "Great Recession Job Losses Severe, Enduring," National Bureau of Economic Research, last updated May 17, 2019, https://www.nber.org/digest/aug15/w21216.html.

20. "Great Recession Job Losses Severe, Enduring."

21. The homeownership rate at ages twenty-five to thirty-four is only 37 percent, compared to 45.4 percent for Gen Xers and 45 percent for baby boomers when they were that age. Jung Hyun Choi, Jun Zhu, and Laurie Goodman, "The State of Millennial Homeownership," *Urban Wire*, July 11, 2018, https://www.urban.org/urban-wire/state-millennial-homeownership.

22. "The Generation Gap in American Politics," Pew Research Center, http://www.people-press.org/2018/03/01/2-views-of-scope-of-government-trust-in-government-economic-inequality.

23. "Freelancing in America, 2017," Edelman Intelligence, September 2017, https://www.slideshare.net/upwork/freelancing-in-america-2017/54.

24. "Contingent and Alternative Employment Arrangements—May 2017," US Bureau of Labor Statistics, June 7, 2018, https://www.bls.gov/news.release/pdf/conemp.pdf; Karen Kosanovich, "Workers in Alternative Employment Arrangements," US Bureau of Labor Statistics, November 2018, https://www.bls.gov/spotlight/2018/workers-in-alternative-employment-arrangements/pdf/workers-in-alternative-employment-arrangements.pdf.

25. David Storey, Tony Steadman, and Charles Davis, *Is the Gig Economy a Fleeting Fad, or an Enduring Legacy?* (Ernst and Young, 2016), https://gigeconomy.ey.com/Documents/Gig%20Economy%20Report.pdf.

26. David Storey, Tony Steadman, and Charles Davis, "How the Gig Economy Is Changing the Workforce," Ernst and Young, 2016, https://www.ey.com/en_gl/tax/how-the-gig-economy-is-changing-the-workforce.

27. Karen Chee, "Freelancers of the World, Unite in Despair!," *New York Times*, October 13, 2018, https://www.nytimes.com/2018/10/13/opinion/sunday/chee-gig-economy-guild-union.html.

28. Storey, Steadman, and Davis, "How the Gig Economy Is Changing the Workforce."

29. Brigitte Madrian, "Employment-Based Health Insurance and Job Mobility: Is There Evidence of Job-Lock?," *Quarterly Journal of Economics* 109, no. 1 (1994): 27–54, doi: 10.2307/2118427.

30. The Consolidated Omnibus Budget Reconciliation Act (COBRA) was passed in 1985 because many people who lost their jobs were simultaneously losing their only means of purchasing health insurance and could be denied coverage because of preexisting conditions. If you quit your job, lose coverage because of reduced hours, or are fired for a reason other than gross misconduct, you can purchase the same plan you had as an employee. However, you have to pay the entire premium without help from the employer, and an extra 2 percent is tacked on for administrative costs. Barbara Marquand, "What you need to know about COBRA insurance," insurance.com, last updated October 23, 2018, https://www.insurance.com/health-insurance/health-insurance-basics/what-you-need-to-know-about-cobra.html.

31. "Real Gross Domestic Product (GDP) of the United States of America from 1990 to 2018 in billion chained (2012) U.S. dollars," Statistica, https://www.statista.com/statistics/188141/annual-real-gdp-of-the-united-states-since-1990-in-chained-us-dollars.

32. "Employer Health Benefits."

33. "Employer Health Benefits."

34. The Trump Administration issued a rule that loosens restrictions on Association Health Plans selling policies, which has the potential to allow small employers and independent contractors to purchase large group plans instead of more strictly regulated small group or individual plans.

35. "Employer Health Benefits."

36. This 1970s experiment randomized families into health plans with different cost-sharing. Some had a "free care" plan with no cost-sharing, and some had a deductible of the equivalent in today's dollars of $6,000; Joseph P. Newhouse, "Consumer-Directed Health Plans and the RAND Health Insurance Experiment," *Health Affairs* 23, no. 6 (2004): 107–13, doi:10.1377/hlthaff.23.6.107.

37. "Employer Health Benefits." In 2018, 58 percent of covered workers had an annual deductible of $1,000 or more for single coverage.

38. Mary E. Reed et al., "In Consumer-Directed Health Plans, A Majority of Patients Were Unaware of Free or Low-Cost Preventive Care," *Health Affairs* 31, no. 12 (2012): 2641–48, doi:10.1377/hlthaff.2012.0059.

39. Rajender Agarwal, Olena Mazurenko, and Nir Menachemi, "High-Deductible Health Plans Reduce Health Care Cost and Utilization, Including Use of Needed Preventive Services," *Health Affairs* 36, no. 10 (2017): 1762–68. doi:10.1377/hlthaff.2017.0610.

40. Cameron Huddleston, "More Than Half of Americans Have Less Than $1,000 in Savings in 2017," GOBankingRates, September 12, 2017, https://www.gobankingrates.com/saving-money/savings-advice/half-americans-less-savings-2017.

41. "Employer Health Benefits." All firms with more than two hundred employees that provide health insurance offer family coverage whereas only 95 percent of firms with fewer than two hundred employees that provide health insurance offer family coverage.

42. "Employer Health Benefits." Employer-sponsored insurance is governed by federal tax and employee benefits law (the Employee Retirement Income Security Act (ERISA)), which supersedes the other laws. Employers' self-insured plans have looser regulations on coverage and are exempt from all state laws governing reserve requirements, mandated benefits, and consumer protections. In terms of essential health benefits, employers are required to cover at least 60 percent of the cost of the ten essential health benefits and must provide "substantial coverage" for inpatient and physician treatment through one of the plans they offer.

CHAPTER 5: THE ACA ONLY GOT US PARTWAY

1. Nancy Pelosi floor speech, American Rhetoric, March 28, 2018, https://american rhetoric.com/speeches/nancypelosihorhealthcarefinalvote.htm.

2. Ashley Kirzinger et al., "Kaiser Health Tracking Poll—March 2018: Non-Group Enrollees," Kaiser Family Foundation, April 10, 2018, https://www.kff.org/health-reform/poll -finding/kaiser-health-tracking-poll-march-2018-non-group-enrollees.

3. This model was designed by Governor Mitt Romney's team during 2005 and was passed into law in 2006. The law, Chapter 58 of the Acts of 2006, was aptly named "An Act Providing Access to Affordable, Quality, Accountable Health Care."

4. Author's presentation delivered March 1, 2010, from Massachusetts Health Connector sources.

5. Rachel Fehr, Cynthia Cox Follow, and Larry Levitt, "Data Note: Changes in Enrollment in the Individual Health Insurance Market through Early 2019," Henry J. Kaiser Family Foundation, August 21, 2019, https://www.kff.org/private-insurance/issue-brief/data-note -changes-in-enrollment-in-the-individual-health-insurance-market-through-early-2019.

6. Kirzinger et al., "Kaiser Health Tracking Poll—March 2018."

7. Michelle Andrews, "Many Individual Health Policies Do Not Cover Pregnancy," Kaiser Health News, November 16, 2010, https://khn.org/news/maternity-expenses.

8. Andrews, "Many Individual Health Policies."

9. Regarding economic tweaking, insurers don't have to outright deny coverage to prevent people from buying a plan. They can simply tweak their plan designs to make them unappealing to undesired enrollees. For example, if a plan doesn't want HIV people to sign up, instead of not allowing them directly they can simply not cover HIV drugs, and HIV-positive people won't purchase the plan. As a result HIV patients end up on some other plan that does cover their drugs, then that plan either loses money or has to drop the drugs to stay afloat.

10. Fearing a race to the bottom and a proliferation of health plans that are useless to anyone with an ongoing condition, the ACA implemented "risk adjustment." Under this program, every single health plan has to send claims data to a federal agency, the Centers for Medicare and Medicaid Services (CMS). CMS then assesses which plans have sicker patients and which have healthier patients and literally takes money away from the plans with healthy people and gives it to plans with sick people, in the exact amounts that CMS's actuaries believe make plans more neutral about how sick or healthy their risk pool is. HIV-positive patients become just as lucrative as enrollees with perfect health.

11. The technical terms for these protections are "guaranteed issue and renewability of health insurance," and no "medical underwriting" (meaning higher premiums) for people with preexisting conditions.

12. "Health Insurance Coverage for Americans with Pre-Existing Conditions: The Impact of the Affordable Care Act," Department of Health and Human Services Office of the Assistant Secretary for Planning and Evaluation, January 5, 2017, https://aspe.hhs.gov/system /files/pdf/255396/Pre-ExistingConditions.pdf.

13. "Health Insurance Coverage for Americans with Pre-Existing Conditions." Before the ACA, these preexisting-condition-coverage limitations applied only to the roughly twelve million people who bought insurance through the individual market. However, that's a misleadingly low number, because millions more were shut out of the markets by the preexisting condition rules or the high prices. And when you consider the people who transition in and out of different types of coverage and the cost to society of lapses in insurance, the true impact was much greater.

14. Gary Claxton et al., "Pre-Existing Conditions and Medical Underwriting in the Individual Insurance Market Prior to the ACA," Henry J. Kaiser Family Foundation, October 12, 2018, https://www.kff.org/health-reform/issue-brief/pre-existing-conditions-and-medical -underwriting-in-the-individual-insurance-market-prior-to-the-aca.

15. Ashley Kirzinger, Bryan Wu, and Mollyann Brodie, "Kaiser Health Tracking Poll— June 2018: Campaigns, Pre-Existing Conditions, and Prescription Drug Ads," Henry J. Kaiser Family Foundation, July 20, 2018, https://www.kff.org/health-costs/poll-finding/kaiser-health -tracking-poll-june-2018-campaigns-pre-existing-conditions-prescription-drug-ads.

16. Hemophilia costs an average of $270,000 per patient per year to treat. Jenny Gold, "Miracle of Hemophilia Drugs Comes at a Steep Price," NPR, March 15, 2018, https://www .npr.org/sections/health-shots/2018/03/05/589469361/miracle-of-hemophilia-drugs-comes -at-a-steep-price.

17. Loren Adler and Paul Ginsburg, "Health Insurance as Assurance: The Importance of Keeping the ACA's Limits on Enrollee Health Costs," Brookings Institution, March 5, 2018, https://www.brookings.edu/blog/usc-brookings-schaeffer-on-health-policy/2017/01/17/health -insurance-as-assurance-the-importance-of-keeping-the-acas-limits-on-enrollee-health-costs. Lifetime limits were common in both the individual and employer health insurance markets before the ACA. In 2009, before the ACA, 59 percent of workers with employer-provided health insurance were in a plan with a lifetime limit on how much it would cover, and 27 percent of those had a lifetime limit between $1 million and $2 million; 89 percent of health plans in the individual market included a lifetime limit, averaging roughly $5 million. "The lifetime cap prohibition is one of the key ways in which the ACA benefits people with employer-provided health insurance, and it represents a valuable gain for many with chronic and catastrophic conditions."

18. Adler and Ginsburg, "Health Insurance as Assurance"; Louise Norris, "ACA Ban on Annual and Lifetime Benefit Maximums Has Caveats," Verywell Health, October 23, 2018, https://www.verywellhealth.com/no-more-lifetime-or-annual-benefit-maximums-but-caveats -apply-1738966.

19. Sarah Kliff, "The Obamacare Provision That Saved Thousands from Bankruptcy," *Vox*, March 2, 2017, https://www.vox.com/policy-and-politics/2017/2/15/14563182/obamacare -lifetime-limits-ban.

20. In fact, a study by PricewaterhouseCoopers found that increasing lifetime limits of a plan from $1 million to $10 million would increase premiums by only about 1 percent. Ken Terry, "No Lifetime Limit on Health Coverage Is A Good Deal for Americans," CBS News, September 23, 2010, https://www.cbsnews.com/news/no-lifetime-limit-on-health-coverage -is-a-good-deal-for-americans.

21. Sarah Kliff, "The AHCA Could Bring Back Lifetime Limits. That's Bad News for This 6-Year-Old Boy," *Vox*, May 4, 2017, https://www.vox.com/policy-and-politics/2017/5/4 /15539010/ahca-lifetime-limits; Alexandra Olgin, "GOP Health Bill Could Let Insurers Cap Spending on Expensive Patients," NPR, June 30, 2017, https://www.npr.org/sections/health -shots/2017/06/30/534773322/gop-health-bill-could-let-insurers-cap-spending-on -expensive-patients.

22. Christopher Warshaw and David Broockman, "G.O.P. Senators Might Not Realize It, but Not One State Supports the Republican Health Bill," *New York Times*, June 14, 2017, https://www.nytimes.com/2017/06/14/upshot/gop-senators-might-not-realize-it-but-not-one -state-supports-the-ahca.html.

23. If well-designed, exchanges could level the playing field for insurers. Small and large insurers can offer products, and no company has an unfair advantage, since wealthier insurers can't buy ads or more space on the website. This keeps things more affordable for consumers, since some smaller insurers have a chance to compete (by bringing more affordable products) that hadn't been available before.

24. Andrew Prokop, "The Battle over Medicaid Expansion in 2013 and 2014, Explained," *Vox*, May 12, 2015, https://www.vox.com/cards/medicaid-expansion-explained.

25. "An Estimated 6.6 Million Young Adults Stayed on or Joined Their Parents' Health Plans in 2011 Who Would Not Have Been Eligible Prior to Passage of the Affordable Care Act," Commonwealth Fund, June 8, 2012, https://www.commonwealthfund.org/press-release /2012/estimated-66-million-young-adults-stayed-or-joined-their-parents-health-plans.

26. Harris Meyer, "Many Consumers Pass Up Premium Subsidies by Buying Off-Exchange Health Plans," Modern Healthcare, August 07, 2017, https://www.modernhealthcare .com/article/20170807/NEWS/170809915/many-consumers-pass-up-premium-subsidies-by -buying-off-exchange-health-plans.

27. Linda Blumberg, Matthew W. Buettgens, and Robin Wang, "The Potential Impact of Short-Term Limited Duration Policies on Insurance Coverage, Premiums, and Federal Spending," Urban Institute, February 2018, https://www.urban.org/sites/default/files/stld _draft_0226_original_0.pdf.

28. Karen Pollitz et al., "Understanding Short-Term Limited Duration Health Insurance," Henry J. Kaiser Family Foundation, April 23, 2018, https://www.kff.org/health-reform /issue-brief/understanding-short-term-limited-duration-health-insurance/?utm_campaign =KFF-2018-April-Health-Reform-Short-Term-Health-Plans&utm_source=hs_email&utm _medium=email&utm_content=2&_hsenc=p2ANqtz-_tvcnVwZyEhL2NsbntoBfiaT8reyBD 7KFEZ6JAmaZSLLXb4uYL8azXlsiwik9vv9ut-9g5OwAvLdFuDF_xhzDYcq1aJA&_hsmi=2.

29. Dylan Scott, "If You Need Prescriptions or Maternity Care, You Won't like Trump's Short-Term Insurance Plans," *Vox*, April 23, 2018, https://www.vox.com/policy-and-politics /2018/4/23/17271798/trump-health-care-prescriptions-maternity.

30. Cheryl Fish-Parcham, "RE: Comments on Short-Term, Limited-Duration Insurance Proposed Rule (CMS-9924-P)," Families USA, April 23, 2018, http://familiesusa.org/sites /default/files/documents/Short-term_health_plan_Families_USA_Comments_4-23-18.pdf.

31. In 2018, the average individual marketplace premium was about $440 per month, with a $4,500 deductible for a single person and $1,200 per month with a $5,900 deductible for families. "How Much Does Obamacare Cost in 2018?," EHealth Insurance Resource Center, June 20, 2018, https://resources.ehealthinsurance.com/affordable-care-act/much-obamacare-cost-2018.

32. Caroline Pearson, Elizabeth Carpenter, and Chris Sloan, "Plans with More Restrictive Networks Comprise 73% of Exchange Market," Avalere Health, October 11, 2018, http://avalere.com/expertise/managed-care/insights/plans-with-more-restrictive-networks-comprise-73-of-exchange-market.

33. Loren Adler and Paul Ginsburg, "Obamacare Premiums Are Lower Than You Think," Health Affairs, July 21, 2016. https://www.healthaffairs.org/do/10.1377/hblog20160721.055898/full.

34. Kirzinger et al., "Kaiser Health Tracking Poll—March 2018."

CHAPTER 6: LEFT UNCOVERED

1. Martin Luther King, "Remarks at the Second Annual Convention of the Medical Committee for Human Rights," speech, Chicago, March 26, 1966.

2. "Health Insurance Coverage of the Total Population," Kaiser Family Foundation, https://www.kff.org/other/state-indicator/total-population/?dataView=1&currentTimeframe=0&sortModel=%7B%22colId%22:%22Location%22,%22sort%22:%22asc%22%7D; Zac Auter, "U.S. Uninsured Rate Steady at 12.2% in Fourth Quarter of 2017," Gallup, January 16, 2018, https://news.gallup.com/poll/225383/uninsured-rate-steady-fourth-quarter-2017.aspx. As noted earlier, the Affordable Care Act did reduce the number of uninsured substantially. Before the ACA went into effect, nearly fifty million Americans were uninsured, but provisions like the Medicaid expansion, the individual marketplaces, and the individual mandate pushed this number down to its current level of twenty-eight million.

3. Auter, "U.S. Uninsured Rate."

4. "Key Facts about the Uninsured Population," Kaiser Family Foundation, https://www.kff.org/fact-sheet/key-facts-about-the-uninsured-population.

5. Ruben Castaneda, "Where Can Undocumented Immigrants Go for Health Care?" *U.S. News and World Report Health*, November 2, 2016, https://health.usnews.com/wellness/articles/2016-11-02/where-can-undocumented-immigrants-go-for-health-care. A study in 2017 found that working-age adults from economically disadvantaged racial groups (black, Hispanic, and Native American) have lower rates of health insurance. *In fact, Hispanics and Native Americans have twice the rate of uninsurance of whites and Asian Americans.* This is partly due to differences in income, immigration status, and structural impediments to coverage. It's also a result of historical barriers that have subjugated minority groups, including the effects of racism. "Uninsured Rates for the Nonelderly by Race/Ethnicity," Kaiser Family Foundation, last updated 2017, https://www.kff.org/uninsured/state-indicator/rate-by-raceethnicity/?currentTimeframe=0&selectedDistributions=white-black-hispanic-asiannative-hawaiian-and-pacific-islander-american-indianalaska-native&sortModel=%7B%22colId%22:%22Location%22,%22sort%22:%22asc%22%7D.

6. Robin Rudowitz et al., "A Closer Look at the Remaining Uninsured Population Eligible for Medicaid and CHIP," Kaiser Family Foundation, February 22, 2016, https://www.kff.org/uninsured/issue-brief/a-closer-look-at-the-remaining-uninsured-population-eligible-for-medicaid-and-chip.

7. "Key Facts about the Uninsured Population."

8. "Key Facts about the Uninsured Population."

9. Kristine Phillips, "'Nobody Dies Because They Don't Have Access to Health Care,' GOP Lawmaker Says. He Got Booed," *Washington Post*, May 7, 2017, https://www.washingtonpost.com/news/powerpost/wp/2017/05/06/nobody-dies-because-they-dont-have-access-to-health-care-gop-lawmaker-says-he-got-booed/?noredirect=on.

10. Woolhandler and Himmelstein, "The Relationship of Health Insurance and Mortality"; "Dying for Coverage: The Deadly Consequences of Being Uninsured," Families USA, June 2012, https://familiesusa.org/sites/default/files/product_documents/Dying-for-Coverage.pdf.

11. "Care Without Coverage: Too Little, Too Late," Institute of Medicine, May 2002, http://www.nationalacademies.org/hmd/~/media/Files/Report%20Files/2003/Care-Without-Coverage-Too-Little-Too-Late/Uninsured2FINAL.pdf.

12. "Care Without Coverage."

13. "Care Without Coverage."

14. "Care Without Coverage."

15. "Care Without Coverage."

16. "Care Without Coverage."

17. Yvonne Gonzalez, "Daughter's Death Drives Nevada Candidate for Congress," *Las Vegas Sun*, May 27, 2018, https://lasvegassun.com/news/2018/may/27/daughters-death-drives-nevada-candidate-for-congre.

18. Amy and Shalynne's story is featured in the documentary *Knock Down the House*, directed by Rachel Lears, Netflix, 2019.

19. In the case National Federation of Independent Businesses (NFIB) v. Sebelius, NFIB was a right-leaning interest group that sued the government in an attempt to dismantle the ACA. Kathleen Sebelius was secretary of Health and Human Services at the time. National Federation of Independent Business v. Sebelius, Secretary of Health and Human Services, 567 U.S. 519 (2012).

20. "Medicaid Expansion & What It Means for You," Healthcare.gov, https://www.healthcare.gov/medicaid-chip/medicaid-expansion-and-you.

21. "Status of State Medicaid Expansion Decisions: Interactive Map," Kaiser Family Foundation, last updated May 13, 2019, https://www.kff.org/medicaid/issue-brief/status-of-state-medicaid-expansion-decisions-interactive-map.

22. "Where Are States Today? Medicaid and CHIP Eligibility Levels for Children, Pregnant Women, and Adults," Kaiser Family Foundation, last updated March 31, 2019, https://www.kff.org/medicaid/fact-sheet/where-are-states-today-medicaid-and-chip.

23. "Where Are States Today?"

24. Remember, the federal poverty level for a single person in 2019 is about $12,500 per year, so this means that any single person living in Texas who earns less than this, or any family of three in Texas who earns between $3,600 and $21,330 in 2019, are ineligible for both Medicaid and individual market subsidies. Without subsidies, any marketplace plan is completely unaffordable for someone with that income. So, they all ended up uninsured.

25. Emily K. Brunson, "'Texans Don't Want Health Insurance': Social Class and the ACA in a Red State," in *Unequal Coverage*, ed. Jessica M. Mulligan and Heide Castañeda (New York: New York University Press, 2018), 185.

26. "eHealth Post-Open Enrollment Report: Premiums Rise Most for Those Under Age 25; Average Family Premium Tops $1,100 Per Month," eHealth, last updated December 20, 2017, https://news.ehealthinsurance.com/news/ehealth-post-open-enrollment-report-premiums-rise-most-for-those-under-age-25-average-family-premium-tops-1-100-per-month.

27. People who don't qualify for subsidies (those who make more than 400 percent of FPL, about $85,000 for a family of three) were originally assumed to earn enough money to purchase an unsubsidized marketplace plan. However, as plan prices rose, coverage became increasingly unaffordable for those making just north of the subsidy cutoff. The average cost of a health plan in 2018 for a family not receiving subsidies was $1,168 per month ($14,000 per year), although prices varied significantly by state. This is a huge increase from what it was in 2014: $667 per month ($8,000 per year). Prices vary by state. "How Much Does Obamacare Cost in 2018?," eHealth, last updated June 20, 2018, https://resources.ehealthinsurance.com/affordable-care-act/much-obamacare-cost-2018.

28. Sarah Kliff, "'Am I a Bad Person?': Why One Mom Didn't Take Her Kid to the ER—Even After Poison Control Said To," *Vox*, May 10, 2019, https://www.vox.com/health-care/2019/5/10/18526696/health-care-costs-er-emergency-room.

29. Commonwealth Fund, "Underinsured Rate Increased Sharply in 2016; More Than Two of Five Marketplace Enrollees and a Quarter of People with Employer Health Insurance Plans Are Now Underinsured," press release, October 18, 2017, https://www.commonwealthfund.org/press-release/2017/underinsured-rate-increased-sharply-2016-more-two-five-marketplace-enrollees-and?redirect_source=/publications/press-releases/2017/oct/underinsured-press-release.

30. "Premiums for Employer-Sponsored Family Health Coverage Rise 5% to Average $19,616; Single Premiums Rise 3% to $6,896," Kaiser Family Foundation, October 3, 2018, https://www.kff.org/health-costs/press-release/employer-sponsored-family-coverage-premiums-rise-5-percent-in-2018.

31. Commonwealth Fund, "Underinsured Rate Increased Sharply in 2016."

32. Cameron Huddleston, "More Than Half of Americans Have Less Than $1,000 in Savings in 2017," GOBankingRates, September 12, 2017, https://www.gobankingrates.com/saving-money/savings-advice/half-americans-less-savings-2017.

33. Samuel L. Dickman, David U. Himmelstein, and Steffie Woolhandler, "Inequality and the Health-Care System in the USA," *Lancet* 389, no. 10077 (2017): 1431–41, doi:10.1016/s0140-6736(17)30398-7; Kim G. Smolderen et al., "Health Care Insurance, Financial Concerns in Accessing Care, and Delays to Hospital Presentation in Acute Myocardial Infarction," *JAMA* 303, no.14 (2010): 1392–1400, doi: 10.1001/jama.2010.409; Huddleston, "More Than Half of Americans."

34. "Underinsured Rate Rose from 2014–2018, with Greatest Growth among People in Employer Health Plans," Commonwealth Fund, February 7, 2019, https://www.commonwealthfund.org/press-release/2019/underinsured-rate-rose-2014-2018-greatest-growth-among-people-employer-health.

35. Commonwealth Fund, "Underinsured Rate Increased Sharply in 2016."

36. "Women's Health Insurance Coverage," Kaiser Family Foundation, last updated December 12, 2018, https://www.kff.org/womens-health-policy/fact-sheet/womens-health-insurance-coverage-fact-sheet.

37. "Women's Health Insurance Coverage."

38. "Women's Health Insurance Coverage."

39. Of underinsured women, 69 percent have problems accessing care because of costs, compared to half (49%) of underinsured men. Commonwealth Fund, "Seven of 10 Women Are Uninsured or Underinsured, Have Medical Bill or Debt Problems, or Problems Accessing Care Because of Cost, New Study Finds," May 11, 2009, https://www.commonwealthfund.org/press-release/2009/seven-10-women-are-uninsured-or-underinsured-have-medical-bill-or-debt-problems.

40. Here are three ways: 1. Although individual plans must cover the ten essential health benefits, one of which is maternity and newborn care, states have the flexibility to select a benchmark plan within that framework, which is further defined by the final rule that CMS releases every year. To offer slightly more affordable products, insurers often try to restrict maternity coverage as much as they can, within the confines of the law, and sometimes even sell plans that violate it. This is done by excluding maternity coverage for dependent enrollees, restricting access to maternity services outside of a plan's service area, and establishing limits on maternity services such as ultrasounds. 2. The Hyde Amendment: Medicaid does not pay for abortions. Also, as of 2019, twenty-six states prohibit exchange plans from covering abortions. 3. Self-insured employer groups have a lot of flexibility regarding which services they cover. In March 2011, in response to objections from religious institutions that did not want to cover contraception, the federal government allowed churches, church associations, parochial schools, and charities (but not hospitals) to refuse to cover contraceptives, even though they are mandated by the ACA. "Women and Health Reform: An Introduction to the

Issues," National Women's Law Center, https://www.nwlc.org/wp-content/uploads/2015/08 /WomenandHealthReform.pdf; "State of Women's Coverage: Health Plan Violations of the Affordable Care Act," National Women's Law Center, https://www.nwlc.org/sites/default /files/pdfs/stateofcoverage2015final.pdf; Alina Salganicoff and Laurie Sobel, "Abortion Coverage in the ACA Marketplace Plans: The Impact of Proposed Rules for Consumers, Insurers and Regulators," Kaiser Family Foundation, last updated December 21, 2018, https://www .kff.org/womens-health-policy/issue-brief/abortion-coverage-in-the-aca-marketplace-plans -the-impact-of-proposed-rules-for-consumers-insurers-and-regulators/; "Insurance Coverage of Contraceptives," Guttmacher Institute, last updated May 1, 2019, https://www.guttmacher .org/state-policy/explore/insurance-coverage-contraceptives.

41. "Health Insurance Coverage of Children 0–18," Kaiser Family Foundation, https:// www.kff.org/other/state-indicator/children-0-18/?dataView=1&currentTimeframe=0&sort Model=%7B%22colId%22:%22Location%22,%22sort%22:%22asc%22%7D.

42. David Brown, Amanda Kowalski, and Ithai Lurie, "Medicaid as an Investment in Children: What Is the Long-Term Impact on Tax Receipts?," National Bureau of Economic Research, Working Paper No. 20835, January 2015, doi:10.3386/w20835.

43. "Children's Health Spending: 2010–2013," Health Care Cost Institute, July 2015, http://www.healthcostinstitute.org/files/HCCI_RB2_0.pdf; "Summary of Pricing Methodology for Accountable Care Organizations and Managed Care Organizations," Massachusetts Executive Office of Health and Human Services, last updated February 7, 2017, https://www .mass.gov/files/documents/2017/02/zw/170208-summary-pricing-methodology-aco-and -mco.pdf?_ga=2.252404809.1543715722.1558031760-768256987.1558031760; Stephen Berman, "Universal Coverage for Children: Alternatives, Key Issues, and Political Opportunities," *Health Affairs* 26, no. 2 (2007): 394–404. doi:10.1377/hlthaff.26.2.394.

44. Samantha Artiga and Petry Ubri, "Key Issues in Children's Health Coverage," Kaiser Family Foundation, last updated February 15, 2017, https://www.kff.org/medicaid/issue-brief /key-issues-in-childrens-health-coverage.

45. "Federal Poverty Level (FPL)," Healthcare.gov, https://www.healthcare.gov/glossary /federal-poverty-level-fpl.

46. Artiga and Ubri, "Key Issues"; Glenn Flores et al., "The Health and Healthcare Impact of Providing Insurance Coverage to Uninsured Children: A Prospective Observational Study," *BMC Public Health* 17, no. 1 (2017), doi:10.1186/s12889-017-4363-z.

47. "Informing CHIP and Medicaid Outreach and Education," Centers for Medicare and Medicaid Services, https://www.insurekidsnow.gov/downloads/campaign/2011-11-topline -survey-findings.pdf.

48. Tricia Brooks et al., "Medicaid and CHIP Eligibility, Enrollment, Renewal, and Cost Sharing Policies as of January 2018: Findings from a 50-State Survey," Kaiser Family Foundation, https://www.kff.org/report-section/medicaid-and-chip-eligibility-enrollment-renewal -and-cost-sharing-policies-as-of-january-2018-findings-from-a-50-state-survey-premiums -and-cost-sharing.

49. CHIPRA also expanded eligibility for CHIP insurance to low-income pregnant women and automatically enrolled newborns when their mothers were eligible for Medicaid or CHIP. It increased funding for outreach and enrollment, offered performance bonuses for states that opted to cover additional children, and streamlined the citizenship verification process to reduce paperwork requirements. "CHIPRA," Medicaid.gov, https://www.medicaid.gov /chip/chipra/index.html; "Express Lane Eligibility for Medicaid and CHIP Coverage," Medicaid.gov, https://www.medicaid.gov/medicaid/outreach-and-enrollment/express-lane/index.html.

50. Tricia Brooks, "States Could Lose Cost-Effective Express Lane Eligibility If Congress Fails to Extend CHIP Promptly," Georgetown University Health Policy Institute, September 13, 2017, https://ccf.georgetown.edu/2017/09/13/states-could-lose-cost-effective-express -lane-eligibility-without-chip-renewal.

51. "State Use of Express Lane Eligibility for Medicaid and CHIP Enrollment," US Office of Inspector General, https://oig.hhs.gov/oei/reports/oei-06-15-00410.asp.

52. Brooks, "State Could Lose."

53. Teresa A. Coughlin et al., "Uncompensated Care for the Uninsured in 2013: A Detailed Examination," Kaiser Family Foundation, https://www.kff.org/uninsured/report /uncompensated-care-for-the-uninsured-in-2013-a-detailed-examination.

54. American Hospital Association, "Uncompensated Hospital Care Cost Fact Sheet," January 2019, https://www.aha.org/system/files/2019-01/uncompensated-care-fact-sheet-jan -2019.pdf.

55. Carlos Dobkin et al., "The Economic Consequences of Hospital Admissions," National Bureau of Economic Research, Working Paper No. 22288, May 2016, doi:10.3386/w22288.

CHAPTER 7: COVERAGE ALONE ISN'T ENOUGH

1. Elizabeth Bradley and Lauren Taylor, *The American Health Care Paradox: Why Spending More Is Getting Us Less* (New York: Public Affairs, 2013), 61.

2. "NCHHSTP Social Determinants of Health," last modified March 10, 2014, Centers for Disease Control, https://www.cdc.gov/nchhstp/socialdeterminants/definitions.html.

3. Sarah Maslin Nir, "Perfect Nails, Poisoned Workers," *New York Times*, May 8, 2015, https://www.nytimes.com/2015/05/11/nyregion/nail-salon-workers-in-nyc-face-hazardous -chemicals.html.

4. Nir, "Perfect Nails."

5. Nir, "Perfect Nails."

6. Nir, "Perfect Nails."

7. Paula Braveman and Laura Gottlieb, "The Social Determinants of Health: It's Time to Consider the Causes of the Causes," *Public Health Reports* 129, no. 1_suppl2 (2014): 19–31, doi: 10.1177/00333549141291S206.

8. "CDC's Anti-Smoking Ad Campaign Spurred Over 100,000 Smokers to Quit; Media Campaigns Must be Expanded Nationally and in the States," Campaign for Tobacco-Free Kids, last modified September 9, 2013, https://www.tobaccofreekids.org/press-releases/2013 _09_09_cdc.

9. Lucie Kutikova et al., "The Economic Burden of Lung Cancer and the Associated Costs of Treatment Failure in the United States," *Lung Cancer* 50, no. 2 (2005): 143–54, doi:10.1016/j.lungcan.2005.06.005.

10. J. Michael McGinnis, Pamela Williams-Russo, and James R. Knickman, "The Case for More Active Policy Attention to Health Promotion," *Health Affairs* 21, no. 2 (2002): 78–93, doi: 10.1377/hlthaff.21.2.78.

11. Room 41 Team, "Crisis Point: The State of Literacy in America," *Room 241: A Blog by Concordia University-Portland*, March 5, 2018, https://education.cu-portland.edu/blog /education-news-roundup/illiteracy-in-america.

12. The Room 41 Team, "Crisis Point."

13. "Assessing Americans' Familiarity with Health Insurance Terms and Concepts," Kaiser Family Foundation, last modified Nov. 11, 2014, https://www.kff.org/health-reform/poll -finding/assessing-americans-familiarity-with-health-insurance-terms-and-concepts.

14. Nancy D. Berkman et al., "Low Health Literacy and Health Outcomes: An Updated Systematic Review," *Annals of Internal Medicine* 155, no. 2 (2011): 97–107, doi: 10.7326/0003 -4819-155-2-201107190-00005.

15. Rebecca L. Sudore et al., "Limited Literacy in Older People and Disparities in Health and Healthcare Access," *Journal of the American Geriatrics Society* 54, no. 5 (2006): 770–76, doi:10.1111/j.1532-5415.2006.00691.x.

16. Saurabh Bhargava, George Loewenstein, and Justin Sydnor, "Choose to Lose: Health Plan Choices from a Menu with Dominated Option," *Quarterly Journal of Economics* 132, no. 3 (2017): 1319–72, doi: 10.1093/qje/qjx011.

17. Glenn Flores, "Language Barriers to Health Care in the United States," *New England Journal of Medicine* 355, no. 3 (2006): 229–31, doi: 10.1056/NEJMp058316.

18. Julianne Holt-Lunstad, Timothy Smith, and J. Bradley Layton, "Social Relationships and Mortality Risk: A Meta-Analytic Review," *PLoS Medicine* 7, no. 7 (2010), doi: 10.1371 /journal.pmed.1000316, https://journals.plos.org/plosmedicine/article?id=10.1371/journal .pmed.1000316

19. Holt-Lunstad et al., "Social Relationships."

20. Chris Crowley and Henry S. Lodge, *Younger Next Year for Women: Live Strong, Fit, and Sexy—Until You're 80 and Beyond* (New York: Workman Publishing, 2007), 311.

21. Crowley and Lodge, *Younger*, 311.

22. Robert Putnam, *Bowling Alone: America's Declining Social Capital* (New York: Palgrave Macmillan, 2000), 331.

23. Atul Gawande, "The Heroism of Incremental Care," *New Yorker*, January 15, 2017, https://www.newyorker.com/magazine/2017/01/23/the-heroism-of-incremental-care.

24. "What is Stigma," Healthy Place for Your Mental Health, last modified July 5, 2016, https://www.healthyplace.com/stigma/stand-up-for-mental-health/what-is-stigma.

25. Philip S. Wang et al., "Failure and Delay in Initial Treatment Contact After First Onset of Mental Disorders in the National Comorbidity Survey Replication," *Archives of General Psychiatry* 62, no. 6 (2005): 603, doi:10.1001/archpsyc.62.6.603.

26. Nancy F. Liu et al., "Erratum: Stigma in People With Type 1 or Type 2 Diabetes," *Clinical Diabetes* 35, no. 4 (2017): 262, doi: 10.2337/cd17-er01.

27. Liu et al., "Erratum."

28. Brett Milano, "African-Americans Say They Are Still Treated Unfairly, Harvard Researchers Find," *Harvard Gazette*, October 30, 2017, https://news.harvard.edu/gazette/story /2017/10/in-new-poll-african-americans-say-they-are-still-treated-unfairly.

29. For an excellent discussion of the effects of unintentional bias and racism, see Robin DiAngelo, *White Fragility: Why It's So Hard for White People to Talk About Racism* (Boston: Beacon Press, 2018).

30. David R. Williams, "Why Discrimination Is a Health Issue," Robert Wood Johnson Foundation, October 24, 2017, https://www.rwjf.org/en/blog/2017/10/discrimination-is-a -health-issue.html.

31. This is sometimes referred to as the "Hispanic health paradox," and it's based on immigration patterns. Although Hispanics tend to be socioeconomically disadvantaged in the US, they are often healthier than their US counterparts. This is because healthy Hispanics living in Latin America are more likely to immigrate to the United States and sicker Hispanics living in the United States are more likely to immigrate to Latin America, and the effects of these immigration dynamics are enough to overcome the effects of income, education, and insurance rates on overall health. Hispanics also have lower smoking rates.

32. Paula A. Braveman et al., "Socioeconomic Disparities in Health in the United States: What the Patterns Tell Us," *American Journal of Public Health* 100, no. S1 (2010), doi: 10.2105 /ajph.2009.166082.

33. Vickie M. Mays, Susan D. Cochran, and Namdi W. Barnes, "Race, Race-Based Discrimination, and Health Outcomes Among African Americans," *Annual Review of Psychology* 58, no. 1 (2007): 201–25, doi:10.1146/annurev.psych.57.102904.190212; David R. Williams, Harold W. Neighbors, and James S. Jackson, "Racial/Ethnic Discrimination and Health: Findings From Community Studies," *American Journal of Public Health* 93, no. 2 (2003): 200–208, doi:10.2105/ajph.93.2.200.

34. Paula Braveman et al., "Housing and Health," Robert Wood Johnson Foundation, https://www.rwjf.org/content/dam/farm/reports/issue_briefs/2011/rwjf70451.

35. Amy Roeder, "Zip Code Better Predictor of Health Than Genetic Code," *Harvard T. H. Chan School of Public Health*, August 4, 2014, https://www.hsph.harvard.edu/news /features/zip-code-better-predictor-of-health-than-genetic-code.

36. "MUA Find," Health Resources & Services Administration, https://data.hrsa.gov /tools/shortage-area/mua-find.

37. Elizabeth L. Tung et al., "Neighborhood Crime and Access to Health-Enabling Resources in Chicago," *Preventive Medicine Reports* 9 (2018): 153–56, doi: 10.1016/j.pmedr .2018.01.017.

38. Rachel L. Carson, Eric Sevareid, and Robert White-Stevens, *CBS Reports*, season 4, episode 14, "The Silent Spring of Rachel Carson," written by Jay McMullen, aired April 3, 1963, on CBS, https://www.imdb.com/title/tt0962224.

39. Libby Nelson, "The Flint Water Crisis, Explained," *Vox*, February 15, 2016, https:// www.vox.com/2016/2/15/10991626/flint-water-crisis.

40. Julia Manchester, "Michigan Congressman Says Flint's Water Still Not Safe to Drink," *Hill*, January 1, 2019, https://thehill.com/hilltv/rising/424536-flints-congressman -says-water-is-still-not-safe-to-drink.

41. "DDT Regulatory History: A Brief Survey (to 1975)," EPA, last modified September 14, 2016, https://archive.epa.gov/epa/aboutepa/ddt-regulatory-history-brief-survey-1975. html; "Health Consequence of Smoking, Surgeon General Fact Sheet," US Department of Health and Human Services, Office of the Surgeon General, last modified January 16, 2014, https://www.surgeongeneral.gov/library/reports/50-years-of-progress/fact-sheet.html.

42. "Protecting the Health of Nail Salon Workers," US Environmental Protection Agency, March 2007, https://www.epa.gov/sites/production/files/2015-05/documents/nail salonguide.pdf.

43. The most commonly cited reason is that Medicaid reimbursement for services is so low that providers lose money caring for these patients. Caregivers also claim that Medicaid patients often have highly complex health problems and that this group creates a considerable administrative burden. Sharon K. Long, "Physicians May Need More Than Higher Reimbursements to Expand Medicaid Participation: Findings from Washington State," *Health Affairs* 32, no. 9 (2013): 1560–67, doi: 10.1377/hlthaff.2012.1010.

44. Hiring, firing, pay, job assignments, promotions, layoff, training, fringe benefits, and any other term of employment cannot be based on disability status. "Disability Discrimination," US Equal Employment Opportunity Commission, https://www.eeoc.gov/laws/types /disability.cfm.

45. Grace Donnelly, "See How Your State Ranks in Employment Among Workers with Disabilities," Fortune.com, February 28, 2017, http://fortune.com/2017/02/28/disability -employment-rank.

46. James A. Morone, *The Devils We Know: Us and Them in America's Raucous Political Culture* (Lawrence: University Press of Kansas, 2014), 103.

47. Morone, *Devils*, 103.

48. Christopher Ingraham, "Wealth Concentration Returning to 'Levels Last Seen During the Roaring Twenties,' According to New Research," *Washington Post*, February 8, 2019, https://www.washingtonpost.com/us-policy/2019/02/08/wealth-concentration-returning -levels-last-seen-during-roaring-twenties-according-new-research/?utm_term=.a6199151c73f.

49. Robert Reich, *The Common Good* (New York: Alfred A. Knopf, 2018), 91.

50. Lauren Carroll, "Hillary Clinton: Top Hedge Fund Managers Make More Than All Kindergarten Teachers Combined," *Politifact*, June 15, 2015, https://www.politifact.com /truth-o-meter/statements/2015/jun/15/hillary-clinton/hillary-clinton-top-hedge-fund -managers-make-more-.

51. Morone, *Devils*, 104.

52. Morone, *Devils*, 139.

53. Sandro Galea, *Well: What We Need to Talk About When We Talk About Health* (New York: Oxford University Press, 2019), 17.

54. Ichiro Kawachi, "Why the United States Is Not Number One in Health," in *Healthy, Wealthy, and Fair: Health Care and the Good Society*, ed. James A. Morone and Lawrence R. Jacobs (New York: Oxford University Press, 2005), 33.

55. Bradley and Taylor, *The American Health Care Paradox*, 98.

56. Kawachi, "Why the United States Is Not Number One in Health," 32.

57. Bradley and Taylor, *The American Health Care Paradox*, 44.

58. Stuart M. Butler, "Social Spending, Not Medical Spending, Is Key to Health," Brookings Institution, July 13, 2016, https://www.brookings.edu/opinions/social-spending -not-medical-spending-is-key-to-health; Jennifer Rubin et al., *Are Better Health Outcomes Related to Social Expenditure?* (Washington, DC: RAND Corporation, 2016), https://www.rand .org/content/dam/rand/pubs/research_reports/RR1200/RR1252/RAND_RR1252.pdf.

59. Bradley and Taylor, *The American Health Care Paradox*, 78

60. "Powering Healthier Communities: November 2010 Community Health Centers Address the Social Determinants of Health," National Association of Community Health Centers, August 2012, http://www.nachc.org/wp-content/uploads/2016/07/SDH_Brief_2012.pdf.

61. Susan Morse, "What Montefiore's 300% ROI from Social Determinants Investments Means for The Future of Other Hospitals," *HealthcareFinance*, July 5, 2018, https://www.health carefinancenews.com/news/what-montefiores-300-roi-social-determinants-investments -means-future-other-hospitals.

62. Virginia Rall Chomitz et al., "A Decade of Shape Up Somerville: Assessing Child Obesity Measures 2002–2011," https://www.somervillema.gov/sites/default/files/shape-up -somerville-bmi-report.pdf; Virginia R. Chomitz et al., "Shape up Somerville: Building and Sustaining a Healthy Community," https://www.somervillema.gov/sites/default/files/shape -up-somerville-story.pdf.

63. Bradley and Taylor, *The American Health Care Paradox*, 2.

64. Mauricio Avendano et al., "Health Disadvantage in US Adults Aged 50 to 74 Years: A Comparison of the Health of Rich and Poor Americans with That of Europeans," *American Journal of Public Health* 99, no. 3 (2009): 540–48, doi: 10.2105/ajph.2008.139469.

65. Bradley and Taylor, *The American Health Care Paradox*, 48.

66. Bradley and Taylor, *The American Health Care Paradox*, 56.

67. Bradley and Taylor, *The American Health Care Paradox*, 183.

CHAPTER 8: SOLUTIONS NEED TO BE POLITICAL, NOT POLARIZING

1. Alice Walker, *Temple of My Familiar* (New York: Harcourt, 1989).

2. Joanne Miller, Jon Krosnick, and Leandre Fabrigar, "The Origins of Policy Issue Salience: Personal and National Importance Impact on Behavioral, Cognitive, and Emotional Issue Engagement," *Political Psychology: New Explorations* (November 10, 2016): 125–71, https://pprg.stanford.edu/wp-content/uploads/The-Origins-of-Policy-Issue-Salience.pdf.

3. Carol Hanisch, "The Personal Is Political: The Women's Liberation Movement Classic with a New Explanatory Introduction," 2006, http://www.carolhanisch.org/CHwritings /PIP.html.

4. Miller, Krosnick, and Fabrigar, "Origins of Policy Issue Salience."

5. Thank you to Professor Jane Mansbridge of the Harvard Kennedy School for the concept of "enlightened preferences."

6. "Political polarization simply measures overlap between the two parties. A high level of political polarization means that Republicans agree with Republicans and that Democrats agree with Democrats." Ezra Klein, "Congressional Dysfunction," *Vox*, May 15, 2015, https://www .vox.com/cards/congressional-dysfunction/what-is-political-polarization.

7. Drew DeSilver, "The Polarized Congress of Today Has Its Roots in the 1970s," Pew Research Center, June 12, 2014, http://www.pewresearch.org/fact-tank/2014/06/12/polarized -politics-in-congress-began-in-the-1970s-and-has-been-getting-worse-ever-since.

8. Klein, "Congressional Dysfunction."

9. For an excellent series on political polarization in the *Washington Post*, start with Nolan McCarty, "What We Know and Don't Know about Our Polarized Politics," *Washington Post*, January 8, 2014, https://www.washingtonpost.com/news/monkey-cage/wp/2014/01/08/what -we-know-and-dont-know-about-our-polarized-politics/?utm_term=.df03ba41fc41.

10. Thomas Mann and Norman Ornstein, "Let's Just Say It: The Republicans Are the Problem," *Washington Post*, April 27, 2012, https://www.washingtonpost.com/opinions/lets

-just-say-it-the-republicans-are-the-problem/2012/04/27/gIQAxCVUIT_story.html?utm _term=.438ad25bd27c.

11. "Trends in Party Affiliation Among Demographic Groups," Pew Research Center for the People and the Press, March 20, 2018, http://www.people-press.org/2018/03/20/1-trends -in-party-affiliation-among-demographic-groups.

12. DeSilver, "The Polarized Congress of Today."

13. Jennifer Tolbert and Larisa Antonisse, "Listening to Trump Voters with ACA Coverage: What They Want in a Health Care Plan," Kaiser Family Foundation, February 22, 2017, https://www.kff.org/health-reform/issue-brief/listening-to-trump-voters-with-aca-coverage -what-they-want-in-a-health-care-plan.

14. Morone and Blumenthal, "The Arc of History."

15. Janie Velencia, "The 2018 Gender Gap Was Huge," FiveThirtyEight, November 9, 2018, https://fivethirtyeight.com/features/the-2018-gender-gap-was-huge.

16. "Is There a Health Care Vote? More for Democrats and Women than Other Groups," Henry J. Kaiser Family Foundation, March 23, 2016, https://www.kff.org/health -reform/press-release/is-there-a-health-care-vote-more-for-democrats-and-women-than -other-groups.

17. This gender gap on healthcare as a priority was most pronounced among Republican and independent voters in 2016: 44 percent of female Republican and 35 percent of female independent voters were more likely to say that healthcare is "extremely important" to their vote for president, compared to 28 percent of male Republican and 26 percent of male independent voters. Among Democratic voters, there was virtually no gender gap: 44 percent of women and 43 percent of men said that healthcare was "extremely important" to their vote for president. "Is There a Health Care Vote?," Kaiser Family Foundation.

18. "Trends in Party Affiliation among Demographic Groups," Pew Research Center.

19. This gender gap is also manifested in presidential voting. Since 1980, women have been more likely to vote Democratic than men are. In the 2016 presidential election, 55 percent of women voted for Hillary Clinton versus 45 percent of men.

20. "U.S. Voter Support For Marijuana Hits New High; Quinnipiac University National Poll Finds 76 Percent Say Their Finances Are Excellent or Good," Quinnipiac University Poll, April 20, 2017, https://poll.qu.edu/national.

21. Richards and Peterson, Make Trouble, 263.

22. "2018 Midterms: Exit Polling," CNN, 2018, https://www.cnn.com/election/2018/exit -polls.

23. Robert Blendon and John Benson, "Public Opinion About the Future of the Affordable Care Act," New England Journal of Medicine 377, no. 9 (August 31, 2017), doi: 10.1056 /nejmsr1710032.

CHAPTER 9: OTHER COUNTRIES LEAD THE WAY

1. "Closing the Gap in a Generation: Health Equity through Action on the Social Determinants of Health. Final Report of the Commission on Social Determinants of Health," World Health Organization, 2008, https://www.who.int/social_determinants/final_report /csdh_finalreport_2008.pdf.

2. T. R. Reid, The Healing of America: A Global Quest for Better, Cheaper, and Fairer Health Care (New York: Penguin Press, 2009), 13.

3. Munira Z. Gunja et al., "What Is the Status of Women's Health and Health Care in the U.S. Compared to Ten Other Countries?," Commonwealth Fund, December 19, 2018, https:// www.commonwealthfund.org/publications/issue-briefs/2018/dec/womens-health-us-compared -ten-other-countries.

4. Reid, The Healing of America, 24.

5. In Britain, hospitals are mostly public and physicians are private (most are not salaried employees—they contract with the NHS). Elias Mossialos et al., "International Profiles of

Health Care Systems," Commonwealth Fund, May 2017, https://www.commonwealthfund
.org/sites/default/files/documents/___media_files_publications_fund_report_2017_may
_mossialos_intl_profiles_v5.pdf.

6. Ruth Thorlby and Sandeepa Arora, "The English Health Care System," Commonwealth Fund, https://international.commonwealthfund.org/countries/england.

7. Reid, *The Healing of America*, 108.

8. Reid, *The Healing of America*, 126.

9. "Both universal hospital insurance (initiated in 1947) and medical care insurance (initiated in 1962) began in Saskatchewan, a prairie province that had elected North America's first
social democratic government in 1944. The adoption of universal hospital insurance was
broadly supported, but state-funded medical insurance emerged from a bitter political struggle culminating in a 23-day doctors' strike that began on the date of implementation." Steven
Lewis, "A System in Name Only—Access, Variation, and Reform in Canada's Provinces," *New
England Journal of Medicine* 372, no. 6 (2015): 497–500, doi: 10.1056/NEJMp1414409.

10. Sara Allin and David Rudoler, "The Canadian Health Care System," Commonwealth
Fund, https://international.commonwealthfund.org/countries/canada.

11. Reid, *The Healing of America*, 73.

12. As of 2016, total contribution was 14.6 percent of wages, with employers and employees each paying 7.3 percent. Miriam Blümel and Reinhard Busse, "The German Health Care
System," Commonwealth Fund, https://international.commonwealthfund.org/countries
/germany.

13. Reinhard Busse et al., "Statutory Health Insurance in Germany: A Health System
Shaped by 135 Years of Solidarity, Self-governance, and Competition," *Lancet* 390, no. 10097
(2017): 882–97, doi: 10.1016/s0140-6736(17)31280-1; Olga Khazan, "What American
Healthcare Can Learn From Germany," *Atlantic*, April 8, 2014, https://www.theatlantic.com
/health/archive/2014/04/what-american-healthcare-can-learn-from-germany/360133/; Richard Knox, "Most Patients Happy with German Health Care," NPR, July 3, 2008, https://
www.npr.org/templates/story/story.php?storyId=91971406.

14. Busse et al., "Statutory Health Insurance in Germany."

15. *Health Care in Germany: The German Health Care System* (Cologne: Institute for Quality and Efficiency in Healthcare, 2018), https://www.ncbi.nlm.nih.gov/pubmedhealth
/PMH0078019.

16. "German Health Care System," Commonwealth Fund.

17. "German Health Care System," Commonwealth Fund.

18. Reid, *The Healing of America*, 233.

19. Sixty percent of Germans say "the system works pretty well and only minor changes
are necessary to make it better," compared to 35 percent of Canadians, 44 percent of British,
and 19 percent of US citizens.

20. Gunja et al., "What Is the Status of Women's Health and Health Care in the U.S.
Compared to Ten Other Countries?"

21. Gunja et al., "What Is the Status of Women's Health and Health Care in the U.S.
Compared to Ten Other Countries?"

22. Reid, *The Healing of America*, 207.

23. Of course, it's difficult to make clean comparisons across countries. Canada does not
spend as much of its GDP on social services as European countries do, and it still has better
health outcomes than the US does. This can be attributed to other factors: healthier lifestyles,
more health coverage, less mass incarceration, less income inequality and race- and income-
based unofficial segregation, and less exposure to environmental pollutants. Support of social
services is also a controversial issue in Canada, with a recent report concluding that Canada
should spend less on health care and more on social services. "Want a Healthier Population?
Spend Less on Health Care and More on Social Services," January 22, 2018, https://www
.eurekalert.org/pub_releases/2018-01/cmaj-wah011618.php.

24. Reid, *The Healing of America*, 215.

25. Surveys show that the only 3 percent of Germans wait over two months to see specialists versus 6 percent of US patients. Germans fare even better on elective surgery: none wait months for elective surgery versus 4 percent of US patients. "Waited Four Months or More for Elective Surgery, 2016," Commonwealth Fund, https://international.commonwealthfund.org/stats/waited_four_months.

26. Bradley and Taylor, *The American Health Care Paradox*, 191.

27. Allen Frances, "We Have Too Many Specialists and Too Few General Practitioners," *Huffington Post*, January 21, 2017, https://www.huffingtonpost.com/allen-frances/we-have-too-many-speciali_b_9040898.html.

28. "Primary Care Workforce Facts and Stats," Agency for Healthcare Research and Quality, last updated July 2018, https://www.ahrq.gov/research/findings/factsheets/primary/pcworkforce/index.html.

29. Isabelle Durand-Zaleski, "The French Health Care System," Commonwealth Fund International Health Care System Profiles, https://international.commonwealthfund.org/countries/france.

30. "Germany: An Overview of the Primary, Secondary and Tertiary Care Structures," TforG, July 6, 2016, https://www.tforg.com/how-we-think/sweetspot-blog/2016/07/06/germany-overview-primary-secondary-tertiary-care-structures.

31. Michael Gmeinder, David Morgan, and Michael Mueller, "How Much Do OECD Countries Spend on Prevention?," OECD Health Working Papers, December 15, 2017, doi: 10.1787/f19e803c-en.

32. Reid, *The Healing of America*, 189.

33. Reid, *The Healing of America*, 185.

34. "Up to 40 Percent of Annual Deaths from Each of Five Leading US Causes Are Preventable," Centers for Disease Control and Prevention, last updated May 1, 2014, https://www.cdc.gov/media/releases/2014/p0501-preventable-deaths.html.

35. Judy Jou et al., "Paid Maternity Leave in the United States: Associations with Maternal and Infant Health," *Maternal and Child Health Journal* 22, no. 2 (2017): 216–25, doi: 10.1007/s10995-017-2393-x.

36. Mauricio Avendano et al., "The Long-Run Effect of Maternity Leave Benefits on Mental Health: Evidence from European Countries," *SSRN Electronic Journal* (2014), doi: 10.2139/ssrn.2436913.

37. *Education Today 2010: The OECD Perspective* (OECD, 2010), 313.

38. "Education Expenditures by Country," National Center for Education Statistics, last updated May 2018, https://nces.ed.gov/programs/coe/indicator_cmd.asp.

39. Alana Semuels, "Good School, Rich School; Bad School, Poor School: The Inequality at the Heart of America's Education System," *Atlantic*, August 25, 2016, https://www.theatlantic.com/business/archive/2016/08/property-taxes-and-unequal-schools/497333.

40. Lilia Vega, "The History of UC Tuition Since 1868," The Daily Clog, May 17, 2009, https://www.dailycal.org/2014/12/22/history-uc-tuition-since-1868; "Tuition and Cost of Attendance," University of California Admissions, http://admission.universityofcalifornia.edu/paying-for-uc/tuition-and-cost/index.html.

41. Anna Bawden et al., "Which Are the Best Countries in the World to Live in If You Are Unemployed or Disabled?," *Guardian*, April 15, 2015, https://www.theguardian.com/politics/2015/apr/15/which-best-countries-live-unemployed-disabled-benefits.

42. Seth A. Berkowitz et al., "Supplemental Nutrition Assistance Program (SNAP) Participation and Health Care Expenditures among Low-Income Adults," *JAMA Internal Medicine* 177, no. 11 (2017): 1642, doi:10.1001/jamainternmed.2017.4841.

43. Ruth Robertson, John Appleby, and Harry Evans, "Public Satisfaction with the NHS and Social Care in 2017," King's Fund, February 28, 2018, https://www.kingsfund.org.uk/publications/public-satisfaction-nhs-2017.

44. "'There Are Some Good Things in Our Health Care System, but Fundamental Changes Are Needed to Make It Work Better,' 2016," Commonwealth Fund, https://international .commonwealthfund.org/stats/fundamental_changes_needed.

45. "'There Are Some Good Things in Our Health Care System,'" Commonwealth Fund.

46. Bradley and Taylor, *American Health Care Paradox*, 194.

CHAPTER 10: EXPANDING HEALTHCARE ACCESS AND AFFORDABILITY

1. Joan Biskupic, "Ginsburg: Court Needs Another Woman," *USA Today*, October 5, 2009.

2. Sara Collins et al., "New Surveys Point to Support for the ACA but Concern Among Enrollees about Its Future," Commonwealth Fund, March 2, 2018, https://www.common wealthfund.org/blog/2018/new-surveys-point-support-aca-concern-among-enrollees-about -its-future.

3. Scott Neuman, "1 in 4 Americans Thinks the Sun Goes around the Earth, Survey Says," NPR, February 14, 2014, https://www.npr.org/sections/thetwo-way/2014/02/14 /277058739/1-in-4-americans-think-the-sun-goes-around-the-earth-survey-says.

4. From 3 to 41 percent, depending on the study. Woolhandler and Himmelstein, "The Relationship of Health Insurance and Mortality."

5. Reid, *The Healing of America*.

6. Frank Newport, "In U.S., Support for Government-Run Health System Edges Up," Gallup, December 1, 2017, https://news.gallup.com/poll/223031/americans-support -government-run-health-system-edges.aspx.

7. "Single-Payer System Definition," Healthinsurance.org, November 10, 2017, https:// www.healthinsurance.org/glossary/single-payer-system. Note: "traditional" Medicare means the non-Medicare Advantage portion of the program (Medicare Advantage is run by private insurers). Also, it does not include the supplemental private insurance that many people pur- chase to cover things that Medicare doesn't.

8. "A Slim Majority of Americans Support a National Government-Run Health Care Program," *Washington Post*, April 21, 2018, https://www.washingtonpost.com/page/2010-2019 /WashingtonPost/2018/04/12/National-Politics/Polling/release_517.xml?tid=a_mcntx.

9. "Public Opinion on Single-Payer, National Health Plans, and Expanding Access to Medicare Coverage," Henry J. Kaiser Family Foundation, June 19, 2019, https://www.kff.org /slideshow/public-opinion-on-single-payer-national-health-plans-and-expanding-access-to -medicare-coverage.

10. Reid, *The Healing of America*, 112.

11. Linda J. Blumberg et al., "Response to Criticisms of Our Analysis of the Sanders Health Care Reform Plan," Urban Institute, May 2016, https://www.urban.org/sites/default /files/publication/80666/2000793-Response-to-Criticisms-of-Our-Analysis-of-the-Sanders -Health-Care-Reform-Plan.pdf.

12. As of mid-2019, the Sanders Medicare for All bill did not include this option.

13. Jan Coombs, *The Rise and Fall of HMOs: An American Health Care Revolution* (Madison: University of Wisconsin Press), 2005.

14. "Timeline: History of Health Reform in the U.S.," Henry J. Kaiser Family Founda- tion, March 25, 2011, https://www.kff.org/wp-content/uploads/2011/03/5-02-13-history-of -health-reform.pdf; Emanuel, *Reinventing*, 136.

15. John Shatto and M. Kent Clemens, "Projected Medicare Expenditures under an Illustrative Scenario with Alternative Payment Updates to Medicare Providers," Centers for Medicare and Medicaid Services Office of the Actuary, June 5, 2018, https://www.cms.gov /Research-Statistics-Data-and-Systems/Statistics-Trends-and-Reports/ReportsTrustFunds /Downloads/2018TRAlternativeScenario.pdf.; Charles Blahous, "How Much Would Medi- care for All Cut Doctor and Hospital Reimbursements?," Economics 21, October 10, 2018, https://economics21.org/m4a-reimbursements-blahous.

16. By Sanders's own optimistic estimates, the cost of single-payer health care with no cost-sharing would be $42 trillion over ten years (an average of $4 trillion per year, including current Medicaid and Medicare spend of $1.3 trillion, so $2.7 trillion in net new spending). Professor Kenneth Thorpe from Emory University estimates the new required revenues for Sanders's plan at $2.4 trillion. The Urban Institute estimates it at $2.5 trillion, and the Committee for a Responsible Federal budget has it at $2.8 trillion. Teresa Ghilarducci, "What Is Medicare for All?" *Forbes*, July 16, 2018, https://www.forbes.com/sites/teresaghilarducci/2018/07/16/what-is-medicare-for-all/#50901589bdob; John Holahan et al., "The Sanders Single-Payer Health Care Plan: The Effect on National Health Expenditures and Federal and Private Spending," Urban Institute, May 9, 2016, https://www.urban.org/research/publication/sanders-single-payer-health-care-plan-effect-national-health-expenditures-and-federal-and-private-spending/view/full_report; Kenneth Thorpe, "Why Sanders's Single-Payer Plan Would Cost More Than His Campaign Says," American Prospect, February 29, 2016, http://prospect.org/article/why-sanders's-single-payer-plan-would-cost-more-his-campaign-says; "Adding Up Senator Sanders's Campaign Proposals So Far," Committee for a Responsible Federal Budget, February 23, 2018, http://www.crfb.org/papers/adding-senator-sanderss-campaign-proposals-so-far.

17. "Current Government Revenue in the US," US Government Revenue, https://www.usgovernmentrevenue.com/total_revenue, accessed September 23, 2019.

18. "FY 2018 Budget in Brief; CMS; Medicare," US Department of Health & Human Services, May 23, 2017, https://www.hhs.gov/about/budget/fy2018/budget-in-brief/cms/medicare/index.html.

19. Author's estimate, which is a rough calculation: the average individual premium is approximately $7,000 per year, multiplied by the number of individuals with employer-sponsored insurance (156 million) equals over $1 trillion per year.

20. Richard Knox, "Why Are U.S. Health Costs the World's Highest? Study Affirms 'It's the Prices, Stupid,'" WBUR, March 13, 2018, https://www.wbur.org/commonhealth/2018/03/13/us-health-costs-high-jha.

21. Other states where single-payer bills have been introduced include Illinois, Maine, Maryland, Massachusetts, Minnesota, Missouri, New Mexico, Oregon, Pennsylvania, Rhode Island, South Carolina, and Washington. "State Single Payer Legislation," Healthcare-Now!, https://www.healthcare-now.org/legislation/state-single-payer-legislation.

22. Jocelyn Kiley, "Most Continue to Say Ensuring Health Care Coverage Is Government's Responsibility," Pew Research Center, October 3, 2018, http://www.pewresearch.org/fact-tank/2017/06/23/public-support-for-single-payer-health-coverage-grows-driven-by-democrats; Juana Summers, "Poll: Most Young Americans Support Government-Run Health Insurance Program," *PBS NewsHour*, October 24, 2018, https://www.pbs.org/newshour/politics/poll-most-young-americans-support-government-run-health-insurance-program.

23. Initial projections put Green Mountain Care's cost at 9.4 percent payroll tax and 3.1 percent income tax, and the savings at 8–12 percent immediately and an additional 12–14 percent over time. John McDonough, "The Demise of Vermont's Single-Payer Plan," *New England Journal of Medicine*, April 23, 2015, doi: 10.1056/NEJMp1501050; Sarah Kliff, "How Vermont's Single-Payer Health Care Dream Fell Apart," *Vox*, December 22, 2014, https://www.vox.com/2014/12/22/7427117/single-payer-vermont-shumlin.

24. "Public Opinion on Single-Payer, National Health Plans, and Expanding Access to Medicare Coverage."

25. Jacob Hacker, "The Road to Medicare for Everyone," *American Prospect*, January 3, 2018, http://prospect.org/article/road-medicare-everyone.

26. Hacker, "The Road to Medicare for Everyone."

27. Linda J. Blumberg, John Holahan, and Stephen Zuckerman, "The Healthy America Program Building on the Best of Medicare and the Affordable Care Act," Urban Institute, May 14, 2018, https://www.urban.org/research/publication/healthy-america-program.

28. Paul Starr, "The Next Progressive Health Agenda," *American Prospect*, March 23, 2017, http://prospect.org/article/next-progressive-health-agenda.

29. Sarah Kliff, "'Medicare at 50': Sen. Debbie Stabenow Explains Her Medicare Buy-In Plan," *Vox*, February 13, 2019, https://www.vox.com/2019/2/13/18220704/medicare-buy-in -universal-coverage-stabenow.

30. Michael Sparer, "'Medicare for All' Is Democrats' New Rallying Cry; 'Medicaid for More' Would Be Even Better," *Vox*, August 23, 2017, https://www.vox.com/the-big-idea/2017 /8/11/16119292/medicare-for-all-medicaid-health-care-expansion.

31. Sparer, "'Medicare for All.'"

32. Carrie Kaufman, "Medicaid Buy-In Goes Down to a Veto," Nevada Public Radio, June 20, 2017, https://knpr.org/knpr/2017-06/medicaid-buy-goes-down-veto.

33. "Schatz, Luján Reintroduce Legislation to Create Public Health Care Option," Brian Schatz, press release, February 14, 2019, https://www.schatz.senate.gov/press-releases/schatz -lujn-reintroduce-legislation-to-create-public-health-care-option.

34. Yuval Rosenberg, "Elizabeth Warren Has New Plan to Improve Health Care—and It Isn't Medicare for All," Fiscal Times, March 22, 2018, http://www.thefiscaltimes.com /2018/03/22/Elizabeth-Warren-Has-New-Plan-Improve-Health-Care-and-It-Isn-t-Medicare -All.

CHAPTER 11: MAKING HEALTHCARE A RIGHT IN THE US

1. Author's conversation with Angela Davis, Radical Commitments Conference, October 29, 2019, Radcliffe Institute.

2. Fifty-eight percent of Americans say it's more important in our society to have the "freedom to pursue goals without state interference," whereas only 38 percent of people in the United Kingdom said this, and even fewer in other European countries. Conversely, only 35 percent of Americans believe that government should "play an active role in society so as to guarantee that nobody is in need," while 55 percent of people in the UK believe this. Richard Wike, "5 Ways Americans and Europeans Are Different," *Fact Tank*, April 19, 2016, https:// www.pewresearch.org/fact-tank/2016/04/19/5-ways-americans-and-europeans-are-different.

3. John Gramlich, "Few Americans Support Cuts to Most Government Programs, Including Medicaid," *Fact Tank*, May 26, 2017, https://www.pewresearch.org/fact-tank/2017 /05/26/few-americans-support-cuts-to-most-government-programs-including-medicaid.

4. Lawrence R. Jacobs, "Health Disparities in the Land of Equality," in Morone and Jacobs, *Healthy, Wealthy, and Fair*, 63.

5. Deborah Stone, "How Market Ideology Guarantees Racial Inequality," in Morone and Jacobs, *Healthy, Wealthy, and Fair*, 66.

6. Myra Strober, "Rethinking Economics Through a Feminist Lens," *American Economic Review* 84, no. 2 (1994): 143–47.

7. Morone, *Devils*, 108.

8. *Report on the Economic Well-Being of U.S. Households in 2017* (Washington, DC: Board of Governors of the Federal Reserve System, 2018), https://www.federalreserve.gov/publications /files/2017-report-economic-well-being-us-households-201805.pdf.

9. Reid, *The Healing of America*, 213.

10. Reid, *The Healing of America*, 219.

11. Gunnar Robert Almgren, *Health Care as a Right of Citizenship: The Continuing Evolution of Reform* (New York: Columbia University Press, 2017), 100.

12. Reid, *The Healing of America*, 186.

13. James A. Morone and Lawrence R. Jacobs, "Introduction: Health and Wealth in the Good Society," in Morone and Jacobs, *Healthy, Wealthy, and Fair*, 8.

14. Mary Gerisch, "Health Care as a Human Right," American Bar Association, https:// www.americanbar.org/groups/crsj/publications/human_rights_magazine_home/the-state-of -healthcare-in-the-united-states/health-care-as-a-human-right.

15. Benjamin I. Page, "What Government Can Do," in Morone and Jacobs, *Healthy, Wealthy, and Fair*, 338.

16. Paul Krugman, "Something Not Rotten in Denmark," *New York Times*, August 16, 2018, https://www.nytimes.com/2018/08/16/opinion/denmark-socialism-fox.html.

17. "A Single Garment of Destiny," Woven, last updated 2019, https://wovenow.org/a-single-garment-of-destiny.

18. Atul Gawande, "Is Health Care a Right?," *New Yorker*, October 2, 2017.

19. Gawande, "Is Health Care a Right?"

20. Bradley and Taylor, *The American Health Care Paradox*, 174.

21. Peter Jacobson and Elizabeth Selvin, "Courts, Inequality and Health Care," in Morone and Jacobs, *Healthy, Wealthy, and Fair*, 235.

22. "IOM Report: Estimated $750B Wasted Annually in Health Care System," Kaiser Health News, September 7, 2012, https://khn.org/morning-breakout/iom-report.

23. Reid, *The Healing of America*, 43.

24. According to the OECD, an average of $1,220 is spent on retail pharmaceuticals per year for each US resident. Canada, the UK, and Denmark pay far less for their drugs, with the UK and Denmark paying less than half of what we pay. If we paid the same amount for drugs as these other nations, we could save upwards of $100 billion per year, possibly up to $200 billion.

25. Daria Pelech, "An Analysis of Private-Sector Prices for Physicians' Services," Congressional Budget Office, January 2018, https://www.cbo.gov/system/files/115th-congress-2017-2018/workingpaper/53441-workingpaper.pdf.

26. Elke Asen, "Top Individual Income Tax Rates in Europe," Tax Foundation, February 22, 2019, https://taxfoundation.org/top-individual-income-tax-rates-europe-2019.

27. Greg Jaffe and Damian Paletta, "Trump plans to Ask for $716 Billion for National Defense in 2019—A Major Increase," *Washington Post*, January 26, 2018, https://www.washingtonpost.com/world/national-security/trump-plans-to-ask-for-716-billion-for-national-defense-in-2019--a-major-increase/2018/01/26/9d0e30e4-02a8-11e8-bb03-722769454f82_story.html?utm_term=.36f5d34b8eda.

28. Craig Whitlock and Bob Woodward, "Pentagon Buries Evidence of $125 Billion in Bureaucratic Waste," *Washington Post*, December 5, 2016, https://www.washingtonpost.com/investigations/pentagon-buries-evidence-of-125-billion-in-bureaucratic-waste/2016/12/05/e0668c76-9af6-11e6-a0ed-ab0774c1eaa5_story.html; Brad Lendon, "What the Massive US Military Budget Pays For," CNN, March 28, 2018, https://www.cnn.com/2018/03/28/politics/us-military-spending-items-intl/index.html.

29. Peter Wagner and Bernadette Rabuy, "Following the Money of Mass Incarceration," Prison Policy Initiative, January 25, 2017, https://www.prisonpolicy.org/reports/money.html; Wendy Sawyer and Peter Wagner, "Mass Incarceration: The Whole Pie 2019," Prison Policy Initiative, March 19, 2019, https://www.prisonpolicy.org/reports/pie2016.html.

30. Lawrence Brown, "Incrementalism Adds Up?" in Morone and Jacobs, *Healthy, Wealthy, and Fair*, 333.

31. Reid, *The Healing of America*, 181.

32. Reid, *The Healing of America*, 182.

33. Bradley and Taylor, *The American Health Care Paradox*, 183.

34. John Thatamanil, "Live Together or Perish Together: Taking a Lesson from Martin Luther King on Election Day," ABC Religion and Ethics, November 6, 2018, https://www.abc.net.au/religion/lesson-from-martin-luther-king-on-election-day/10469110.

35. Thank you, Senator Cory Booker, for these inspirational ideas.

CHAPTER 12: THE ACTIVISM AGENDA

1. Rosa Parks, *Dear Mrs. Parks: A Dialogue with Today's Youth* (New York: Lee & Low Books, 1996), 87.

2. Marie Gottschalk, "Organized Labor's Incredible Shrinking Social Vision," in Morone and Jacobs, *Healthy, Wealthy, and Fair*, 154.

3. John E. McDonough, *Inside National Health Reform* (Berkeley: University of California Press, 2011), 95.

4. Cayden Mak, "What Happens Next," 18 Million Rising, May 2, 2017, https://18 millionrising.org/2017/01/inauguration.html.

5. Leo Eisenstein, "To Fight Burnout, Organize," *New England Journal of Medicine* 379, no. 6 (2018): 509–11, doi: 10.1056/nejmp1803771.

6. I encourage all who are interested in learning more about the personal benefits and political power of activism to read Richards and Peterson, *Make Trouble*, and *My Life on the Road*, by Gloria Steinem (New York: Random House, 2015). In addition, Angela Davis provides inspiring words of wisdom in her talks and interviews. See, Angela Davis, "Social Justice," interviewed by Common, UCLA Social Justice Summit, C-SPAN, January 12, 2019, https://www.c-span.org/video/?456737-1/angela-davis-common-ucla-social-justice-summit.

7. Steinem, *My Life on the Road*, 129.

8. Gretchen Rubin, *The Happiness Project* (New York: HarperCollins, 2009), 141.

9. Debra Meyerson, "Radical Change the Quiet Way," *Harvard Business Review*, October 2001.

10. Traister, *Good and Mad*, 209.

11. Traister, *Good and Mad*, 234.

12. Morone and Jacobs, *Healthy, Wealthy, and Fair*, 350.

13. Beatrix Hoffman, "Health Care Reform and Social Movements in the United States," *American Journal of Public Health* 93, no. 1 (2003): 7585, doi:10.2105/ajph.93.1.75.

14. Brown, "Incrementalism," 332. Since voter turnout is much higher among high-income people (86 percent) than it is for low-income people (52 percent), higher income people have a disproportionate voice in politics, through their votes as well as their donations.

15. David Wilson and Paul Brewer, "Healthcare Law Gender Gap," *Newswise*, June 26, 2012, https://www.newswise.com/articles/healthcare-law-gender-gap.

16. "'I'm Betting My Life on It': Prof. Gunnar Almgren on Health Care Reform," Center for Human Rights, University of Washington, September 12, 2017, https://jsis.washington .edu/humanrights/2017/09/12/health-care-as-a-right-of-citizenship.

17. Marshall Ganz and Hahri Han, "What Hillary Clinton Can Learn from Bernie Sanders and Donald Trump," *Nation*, June 22, 2016, https://www.thenation.com/article/what-hillary -clinton-can-learn-from-bernie-sanders-and-donald-trump.

18. Sarah Kliff, "The Research Is Clear: Electing More Women Changes How Government Works," *Vox*, March 8, 2017, https://www.vox.com/2016/7/27/12266378/electing -women-congress-hillary-clinton.

19. Author's conversation with John McDonough, November 2018. McDonough noted that we need both types of activism from social movement theory: Saul Alinsky's "brick by brick" approach and Frances Fox Piven's "explosion"—these attract two different types of people to the work.

20. Jeanne Lambrew and Ellen Montz, "The Next Big Thing in Health Reform: Where to Start?," *American Prospect*, January 2, 2018, http://prospect.org/article/next-big-thing-health -reform-where-start.

21. "10 Essential Health Benefits Bill Passes the House," Connecticut House Democrats, http://www.housedems.ct.gov/10-Essential-Health-Benefits-Bill-Passes-the-House; Russell Blair, "9 New Connecticut Laws That Begin on Jan. 1," *Hartford Courant*, January 1, 2019, https://www.courant.com/politics/hc-pol-connecticut-new-laws-january-20190101-5omtjky 3cvcthh2h3qjbx3d6zy-story.html.

22. "Status of State Medicaid Expansion Decisions: Interactive Map," Kaiser Family Foundation, May 13, 2019 https://www.kff.org/health-reform/slide/current-status-of-the -medicaid-expansion-decision.

23. "Where the States Stand on Medicaid Expansion: 36 States, D.C., Have Expanded Medicaid," Advisory Board, April 1, 2019, https://www.advisory.com/daily-briefing/resources /primers/medicaidmap.

24. Bradley and Taylor, *The American Health Care Paradox*, 196.

25. Daniel Victor, "Here's Why You Should Call, Not Email, Your Legislators," *New York Times*, November 22, 2016, https://www.nytimes.com/2016/11/22/us/politics/heres-why-you -should-call-not-email-your-legislators.html.

26. Rowe-Finkbeiner, *Keep Marching*.

AFTERWORD

1. Sonia Sotomayor, *My Beloved World* (New York: Alfred A. Knopf, 2013), 115.

2. Daryl Lindsey, "A Beginners Guide to Activism: 10 Ways to Get Involved with Issues that Matter," *The Everygirl*, February 7, 2017, https://theeverygirl.com/a-beginners-guide-to -activism-10-ways-to-get-involved-with-issues-that-matter.

3. Steinem, *My Life on the Road*.

4. Rowe-Finkbeiner, *Keep Marching*.

GLOSSARY

1. James K. Elrod and John L. Fortenberry, "Centers of Excellence in Healthcare Institutions: What They Are and How to Assemble Them," *BMC Health Services Research* 17, no. 1 (2017): 425, doi: 10.1186/s12913-017-2340-y.

2. Commonwealth Fund, "Underinsured Rate Increased Sharply in 2016."

INDEX

abolition of slavery, 26, 27
abortions, 17, 33, 205n40
ACA. *See* Affordable Care Act (ACA)
activism. *See* women's activism in healthcare reform
ACT UP, 26
adverse selection, 14
affordability: of healthcare system, 3, 21, 61, 62–63, 64; of health coverage, 61, 63–65, 204n27. *See also* economic considerations
Affordable Care Act (ACA): activism on defending, 23–24, 33–34, 171–72, 175–76; on annual or lifetime benefit caps, 57–58; attempts to repeal, 3, 62, 203n19; cost containment provisions in, 58–59, 145; essential health benefits of, 54–56; establishment of, 3–4, 10–11, 16–17; exchange plans of, 44, 59–60, 63, 138; on fair pricing, 58; individual mandate coverage of, 9, 19, 53–54, 62–63; Massachusetts model and, 49–52, 59; need for, 14–16; Pelosi on, 10, 17–18, 49, 144, 166; political polarization and, 18–19, 104–8, 194n17; on preexisting conditions, 9, 56–57, 144; shortcomings of, 59, 61–62, 70–74, 144–45; strengths of, 143–44
African Americans: abolition of slavery, 26, 27; health effects of racism towards, 87–89, 93; uninsurance of, 88, 202n5; voting affiliation of, 108; women's health activism by, 28–31, 32. *See also* black women
AIDS activism, 26, 67. *See also* HIV/AIDS
AKA Mississippi Health Project, 29

Alabama, 71
Alaska, 176
Almgren, Gunnar, 173
ambulatory (outpatient) services, 54, 55, 188
American Association for Labor Legislation, 27
American Association of Retired Persons (AARP), 140
American Cancer Society, 28
American culture and values, 129, 148–56, 215n2
American Health Care Act (2017), 58
The American Health Care Paradox (Bradley and Taylor), 97, 156
American Indians, 88, 93, 202n5. *See also* women of color
American Medical Association, 11, 135, 172
American Medical Student Association, 172
anger, 34–35, 169
annual benefit caps, 57–58
antismoking campaign, 83, 92
Arizona, 13
Arrow, Kenneth, 132
asthma, 82
asymmetric polarization, 104. *See also* partisan politics

Bane, Mary Jo, 110–11
bankruptcy from medical care events, 4, 14, 78. *See also* debt from medical expenses; economic considerations
Baucus, Max, 194n17
Baylor Hospital, 40–41
Beaton, Robin, 15–16
Beveridge, William, 113

ABOUT THE AUTHOR

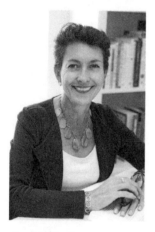

Rosemarie Day is the founder and CEO of Day Health Strategies, where she focuses on implementing national health reform and transforming the healthcare system. She's been working in healthcare and public service for more than thirty years, including as the founding deputy director and chief operating officer of the Health Connector in Massachusetts, where she helped launch the award-winning organization that established the first state-run health insurance exchange in the United States. She also served as the chief operating officer for the Massachusetts Medicaid program. Rosemarie lives with her family in Somerville, Massachusetts. This is her first book.